Yoga and the Five Elements

Yoga and the Five Elements presents a depth of understanding of the subtle elements of the universe that often lie unseen in everyday life. Beyond a yoga practice guide or a philosophical discourse, it presents clear and accessible techniques for anyone yearning to take a journey of reshaping and balancing body, mind, and heart. The reader is guaranteed to reap a harmonious and meaningful connection with nature, oneself, and others. An enriching guide that you'll come back to time and again.
Liz Owen, author of *The Yoga Effect: A Proven Program for Depression and Anxiety*

Yoga and the Five Elements is a thoughtful and accessible guide to living in greater balance, connection, and harmony with ourselves, others, and the world we share. Reflecting the light of Yoga psychology through the lens of modern Theosophy, the book shines its timeless wisdom and healing arts on the complex challenges of our daily lives, using the simple teaching of the five elements to bring it all down to earth. If you're looking for a full tool-kit of insights and practices you can apply right now, you'll want to read this book.
Joseph J. Loizzo, MD, PhD, author of *Sustainable Happiness: The Mind Science of Well-Being, Altruism, and Inspiration*

After 14 years of studying Vedanta, I, an Indian, crossed paths with Nicole Goott, an American, whose depth and understanding of Buddhism, Vedanta, Yoga Shastra together with Western Philosophies left me in awe. Her book *Yoga and the Five Elements* not only reinforced my assimilation of Vedanta but also layered it with Western thought in a very profound and integrated manner. The Mahatattvas or the 5 elements, together with the 3 Gunas, can very well be termed as the tangible starting point of Creation. Debates abound, but if we circle back to the current moment of our primary as well as primal interest in ourselves, i.e. the well-being of our 5 bodies, then it goes right back to the starting point — the 5 tattvas and the 3 gunas — and our need to balance and align them so that we attain the harmony we are perpetually seeking.

This is Nicole's achievement in this book. A calm, mature and logical approach to the practices that balance the elements — in nature and in us — so that everything that we see as 'other' gets dissolved into Oneness.

A must-read for anyone invested in their health, happiness, and well-being.

Neeru Nanda, Seeker & Writer, author of *If: A Collection of Short Stories*

Yoga and the Five Elements

Spiritual Wisdom for Everyday Living

Yoga and the Five Elements

Spiritual Wisdom for Everyday Living

Nicole Goott

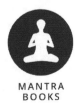

MANTRA
BOOKS

Winchester, UK
Washington, USA

JOHN HUNT PUBLISHING

First published by Mantra Books, 2023
Mantra Books is an imprint of John Hunt Publishing Ltd., No. 3 East Street, Alresford
Hampshire SO24 9EE, UK
office@jhpbooks.com
www.johnhuntpublishing.com
www.mantra-books.net

For distributor details and how to order please visit the 'Ordering' section on our website.

ISBN: 978 1 80341 267 2
978 1 80341 268 9 (ebook)
Library of Congress Control Number: 2022944360

A CIP catalogue record for this book is available from the British Library.

Design: Lapiz Digital Services

UK: Printed and bound by CPI Group (UK) Ltd, Croydon, CR0 4YY
Printed in North America by CPI GPS partners

We operate a distinctive and ethical publishing philosophy in
all areas of our business, from our global network of authors to
production and worldwide distribution.

Contents

O Hidden Life, vibrant in every atom;
O Hidden Light, shining in every creature;
O Hidden Love, embracing all in Oneness;
May all who feel themselves as one with Thee,
Know they are therefore one with every other.
Annie Besant

Preface

About thirteen years ago, I was living in a condo in the city of Boston. My neighbors at the time, who lived across the hall from me, had invited me over to visit. I quickly learned that instead of putting up a bookshelf and filling it with actual books, they had instead painted a bookshelf onto a large span of their living room wall. Like other visitors to their apartment, I was invited to imagine myself as an author. I was invited to paint "my book" that I had "published" into their imaginary library, either fiction or non-fiction. So I thought, why not, and added my name and a book title to a shelf. I had all but forgotten about that experience until now. Looking back on that experience, I can see how it was possibly an early seed for becoming a writer. I've been on a spiritual journey for more than thirty years, and in that time, I've had an opportunity to discover and synthesize teachings and practices that lead to an experience of joyful living. Spiritual teachings found in Indian philosophy have particularly resonated with me. What began as early childhood wonderings has become a lifelong pursuit of the spiritual life and, eventually, a calling to teach. As a young child, I remember wondering to myself, *who am I, where am I?*, questions that human beings for eons have wrestled with. We may not all be drawn to a contemplative life, but across the planet, every individual has a desire to live a fulfilling, peaceful, and joyful life with all their basic needs being met. The way toward these desires being fulfilled means different things to different people. Naturally, I believe this leads to the question – how do we human beings balance our personal needs with everyone else's needs? This question drives a core theme in the book: discovering a way to live harmoniously.

I had begun to explore this idea in classes and workshops that I had been teaching, the focus of which was self-development, geared toward students of yoga but open to spiritual seekers in general. Around the same time, I was attending the spiritual orienteering classes of my long-time spiritual teacher, Kurt Leland. Under the guidance of Kurt, and his inner teacher referred to as *Charles*, the classes deftly explore the inner dimensions of consciousness and energy. In this particular series, we were examining ways in which our energy was balanced or imbalanced from the perspective of the elements of earth, water, air, and fire. The classes highlighted a special interest I'd had along these lines, especially as it related to the origins of the five elements within Indian philosophy. Coupled with my love for Nature and the beings that inhabit it, it seemed obvious to me that a spiritual framework of human self-development would include our shared relationship with Nature. As the book began to evolve, it became clearer to me that I could present a model for spiritual and self-development that would appeal not only to students of yoga but also to contemporary spiritual seekers, who would be interested in tools for spiritual growth. I also believed it was possible to highlight that we're far more similar and connected than we are different and separate. The book, therefore, seeks to outline a spiritual framework and model for balanced and harmonious living derived from the five elements of Nature: earth, water, air, fire, and space. I've outlined a series of practices in each chapter to bring the concepts alive into daily exercises that are accessible. These practices help you find and eventually sustain a more joyful and balanced life.

When it comes to a spiritual path, there is no *right way*. The path that is right for me may not be right for you. I present *a view* within the book, but it is certainly *not the only* view. As you travel with me, I encourage you to consider the following questions:

1. Are the views in the book in conflict or agreement with your core values?

2. What new perspectives develop within you from reading this book?

3. Does the book offer you a new way of seeing yourself and others with more compassion?

The Buddha famously taught that no student should blindly accept his teachings. He wisely asked followers to balance the trust placed in the guidance of an external authority with the wisdom and discernment of their inner authority. An inner teacher exists within all of us. I hope that this book may connect you more deeply with your inner teacher and that whatever resonates for you touches your heart.

Any interpretations, understandings, and errors in this book are my own. It is my humble hope that the book contributes in some way to a more joyful and harmonious union for all beings.

Acknowledgements

I don't think there was ever a time when I considered that I would actually write a book. There may have been occasional musings, wondering a few "what if" scenarios in my mind. Still, the actual process of writing a complete book seemed more wishful than an actual possibility realizing itself. As I reflect on what is needed for someone to write a book, I believe two things need to be present: time and support. I am incredibly fortunate that both of these showed up in abundance in the time in which this book unfolded.

My first debt of gratitude is for my husband, without whom I would not have had the strength nor courage to continue, especially on the days when self-doubt or other worries would assail my mind. You gave me the permission I could not quite give myself on my own to step back from what I was doing in order to wholly dedicate myself to producing my first book.

For my parents, not only for creating the conditions for my entry into this world but also for the enduring and constant love, support, and encouragement to pursue my dreams, including those that involved my moving across many oceans. You will always be my first and best life cheerleaders.

Writing this book synthesizes many of the concepts, beliefs, and practices I have studied formally and informally for the past twenty years. The inspiration, and impetus for bringing it all together, is rooted in a series of meditation classes with Kurt Leland. He is an inspiring author, teacher, and channel whom I have had the great fortune of knowing for the past ten years. The classes provided the missing link, uniting an agglomeration of earlier concepts into a meaningful and useful framework. I am eternally grateful for the kindness, friendship, book coaching, and deep wisdom you have lovingly and unselfishly given.

I have learned that you become a teacher when there are students to teach. For all the wonderful students that have entrusted me over the years, bringing me into your hearts and minds, and giving me the opportunity to learn along with you, thank you. Each time you showed up, you challenged me to grow, and it is through those moments I have continued to learn what it means to teach others.

For all the teachers, both embodied and non-physical, whose faith in me, words of encouragement, or support, thank you. Your showing up provided a rope that I have been able to climb so that I could reach where I am today.

It has been a leap of faith to undertake the project of writing a book. For all the friends, family, former students, and teachers who have generously been willing to read the first tentative pages and early drafts of the manuscript, I am eternally grateful. Holly, Sue, and Sarah, thank you.

Many teachers have generously shared their time and knowledge in the books that they have written. Their books over the years have been steady companions, personal tutors in a way. Other books were of great assistance to me as I wrote my own. To all the teachers whose wisdom has supported me, thank you.

Going into a bookstore, a favorite pastime of mine, one rarely, if ever, considers what it took for all those books to get themselves onto the shelves. The world of publishing is varied, including the option to self-publish, a tool more readily available to writers today than in previous decades. With caring, support, encouragement, and a willingness to share their own experience, I am thankful to Covie for sharing her time, exuberance, and enthusiasm.

In the course of this book being accepted for publication, I joined a marvelous organization for writers – the Society of Authors. I received incredibly thorough and instructional guidance from Elizabeth Haylett Clark which proved to be an invaluable gift. For her time and support, I am immensely grateful.

Writing a book is certainly not a race, but a component of steady endurance is needed, much like a marathon runner. As I neared the completion of writing the book, I had the opportunity to travel, an accomplishment itself amidst a global pandemic. I met some wonderful individuals along the way. They were like the fans cheering the runners to keep going in their final stretch alongside the road. To these individuals, please know that you provided invaluable enthusiasm and encouragement right when it was needed most.

To all those whom I have not named and thanked individually, please know that you are part of a larger community that I hold in my heart with enduring gratitude and love.

Note on Sanskrit and transliteration

Vedic scripture is written in the ancient language of Sanskrit, a language that traces its origins to Southern Asia. There are forty-nine letters in the alphabet, using diametrical marks which accent the letters, and indicate where annunciation and intonation is emphasized. Languages such as English, do not utilize a system of diacritical marks, thus making an equivalent one to one translation not entirely accurate. Translating any language from one system to another is not without its challenges, in particular where original meaning and context can easily be lost in that translation process. In order to account for this in the Sanskrit language, a transliteration scheme emerged, facilitating the movement between languages with greater ease. In simple terms, it works by swapping one set of letters or characters from one language to another language in a predictable schema. The transliteration scheme is a recognized standard called 'The International Alphabet of Sanskrit Transliteration' or IAST.

I have attempted to honor this transliteration system that makes it possible to read a Sanskrit word in English. For example, *kośa* is the Sanskrit word for a non-physical layer or cloak surrounding the individual physical body. It is pronounced *kosha*, emphasizing the "k" as in the word "kick." The "sh" makes the sound similar to the word "wish."

The first time a Sanskrit word appears in the book, it is written in the IAST format with the diacritical marks. Thereafter, the term is written in the Romanized form without the diacritical marks. Further examples include *Śiva* (written as Shiva), *Śakti* (written as Shakti), and *kleśa* (written as klesha). In some instances, however, a word such as *kośa* will form part of a term appearing for the first time in the book, such as *Annamaya kośa*. In this instance, the IAST format will be used. At times

7

throughout the book, to preserve the source material quoted from other authors, I have reproduced the text as it was written.

Any errors or omissions in transliteration are the author's own.

Introduction

Human beings by nature seek meaning in all that they experience. There is a shared fundamental curiosity, a desire to learn, to understand, and to know. Whilst the views may vary, all traditions and religions share an underlying structure that provides a view around which individuals may orient themselves for a sense of direction. If you've ever found yourself lost going anywhere, like the mundane trip to the grocery store in your new neighborhood; direction is only one part of successful navigation. A map is needed, and with it, understanding how to use that map. This book is not going to teach you how to use a printed map or phone app to buy groceries, but it may offer a framework for inner guidance, a journey, and a quest to the very heart of the true Self.

As a meta-framework, the five elements of earth, water, fire, air, and space are easily recognizable as forces existing around us all the time. As with the axiom, we are a microcosm of a larger macrocosm, this is true of the five elements existing not only around us in the Natural world but also within us, in both physical and metaphysical terms.

I was first exposed to the ideas of a five-element theory during my teenage years. My father had practiced Karate for some time, and eventually, I took up the practice of the martial art Kung Fu; and later Tai Chi. One of the primary lessons in the practice, particularly in Tai Chi, involves the ability to harness one's own energy, called *Chi*. Stagnant or blocked energy could be traced back to an imbalance with one or more of the five elements. In Chinese philosophy, they are earth, water, metal, fire, and wood. The healing modality of acupuncture is one system that aims to rebalance blocked energy through the use of small needles inserted into various nexus points along meridian pathways.

I found many similarities when I began to learn about Ayurveda and then, Hatha Yoga. For instance, Hatha Yoga teaches specialized techniques such as breathing practices called *prāṇāyāma* (control or restraint of breath or life force), which seek to control and manipulate unseen energy called *prāṇa* (life force). Ayurveda (a healing modality originating in one of the branches of Indian philosophy) on the other hand seeks to restore and maintain balance through the application of lifestyle changes (diet, daily routines, meditation, etc.), body therapies such as detoxification and massage, herbal remedies, mantra, astrology, and the use of gems.

Despite all my studies, my curiosity and yearning remained unsatisfied. Thus, I continued in my efforts to trace the origins of a five-element theory within Indian philosophy. My intention in writing the book is not to present a historically researched evolution and influence of the five elements as it appears in Yoga today, but to share the synthesis that I have found and how it can be applied to daily living. And, within this synthesis, I also feel that it would be incomplete to not at the very least, reflect upon some of the origins of a framework that I believe has importance and relevance for today. In what has felt a little like falling down a rabbit hole, it remains unclear to me at the time of this writing, how the concept of this fivefold framework evolved over the centuries through the literature of Indian philosophy. The field of research into the ancient texts of Vedic literature is continuing to expand, with growing efforts to translate a vast body of writing for further study and reflection. It's too broad a subject for this book to examine the variations, compilations and adaptations that have occurred throughout the history of Vedic literature and yoga as we know it today.

To honor this effort, one such body of literature in which the ideas of a cosmic and human framework based on the five elements can be found in one of the twelve sutras within the

Taittirīya Upanishad. Swami Satyananda Saraswati translates lesson seven to read:

> *One should meditate upon the elements of which this whole universe is constructed, namely, earth, sky, heaven, the primary and intermediate quarters, fire, air, the sun, the moon, stars, water, herbs, trees, ether and the body. Then again one should meditate upon oneself, considering prana, vyana, apana, udana and samana, the organs of sight, hearing, thinking, speech and the sense of touch, and skin, flesh, muscles, bones and marrow. Having revealed thus by intuition, the seer proclaimed that the whole universe is based on verily this fivefold principal, and one set of five fulfills the other.*
> (Saraswati, 2004, p. 223)

While Ayurveda is said to have its origins within the four Vedas (Rig-Veda, Atharva-Veda, Yajur-Veda, Sāma-Veda), it was eventually expounded upon and edited in what is known as the Caraka Samhitā (Indian Traditional Medicine). Veda is a Sanskrit word that is usually translated to mean a source of sacred knowledge. As a source and collection of many different spiritual worldviews, Vedic literature is composed of a vast range of teachings that evolved from four primary branches. One of those branches produced a set of texts called the Upaniṣads, totaling approximately one hundred and eight, and each varying in length. Each Upanishad is written as a concatenation of *sūtras*. A sutra is an aphorism or short statement which, when woven together, forms something like a tapestry, each verse connected to form a complete idea. A system of healing, Ayurveda maintains that an individual can be perceived as constituting physical and subtle properties. This is conceptualized as a model of three bodies: i) the Gross body (*Shtūla Sharīra*), ii) the Astral body (*Linga Sharīra*), and iii) the Causal body (*Kārana Sharīra*). The bodies are made up of the five elements, further conceptualized as subtle layers called the *kośas* (pronounced "kosha"; meaning a sheath or cloak). Not limited to the individual, the Universe itself is conceived of as being constructed of the five elements; a view that is consistent with the philosophy of *Sāṁkhya*. Interestingly, according to a 2016 NCBI paper, researchers suggest: "Ayurveda has its foundations laid by the ancient schools of Hindu Philosophical teachings named Vaisheshika and the school of logic named as Nyaya" (Jaiswal and Williams, 2016). These philosophical teachings, namely Vaisheshika, can be found in the *Vaiśeṣikasūtra*.

In a later development, the Tantric views found in the Shaivite traditions of Kashmir, built upon the earlier *Sāṁkhya* system and theory of the universe. Samkhya proposed a dualistic version of reality, based on twenty-four cosmic principles with the Absolute or Brahma as a superimposition onto the world as an illusion. Tantra, on the other hand, expanded the cosmic principles in number to thirty-six. Here, the Absolute as Brahma is seen as part of the world illusion in which Brahman has projected itself into the world. This is essentially a non-dual view of the ultimate reality. While there may be some differences, the systems are more complementary than not. Both share a similar perspective wherein the five elements form part of the creation process in which the true Self is veiled in ever-increasing subtlety.

As yoga was developing in the West in the nineteenth century, many of its ideas were being brought over by various teachers such as the well-known Swami Vivekananda who spoke at the first Parliament of the World's Religions in Chicago in 1893. These ideas already had a foothold before some of the more well-known teachers came to the West. In 1875, Madame H.P. Blavatsky founded the Theosophical Society, an endeavor bridging the ideas of Eastern and Western thinking within a framework supported by the value of a brotherhood of all humanity. The Theosophical Society has had a lasting impact on the transmission of these ideas, bridging together east and west. One of these bridges builds upon the koshas, for instance using the term *subtle body* instead of *sheath* which, as Annie Besant says, is "putting together the two ways of looking at the same thing" (Besant, A. 1994, p. 194). It's interesting to note this evolution in nomenclature, I believe, as it offers us insight into how systems can be changed and adapted over time. Annie Besant, like her teacher, H.P. Blavatsky, was interested in presenting spiritual teachings and philosophies in a way that was simple, clear, and easy to relate to for her students. From the point of view for constructing a useful cosmic and self-development framework, Annie Besant offers us, I believe, a useful template. It should be clear, simple, and true. These principles together with the five elements as a framework, have become an essential foundation of my daily life and personal spiritual practice. In the book, I have tried to simplify the concepts, providing what I hope is an approachable and accessible framework. I have chosen to use the nomenclature *subtle body*, which includes the concepts of a subtle layer or sheaths as it may have been conceived of in early Indian philosophy. The book seeks to answer three central questions from the view of the five elements and the subtle bodies as vehicles for consciousness:

1. What is the nature of our reality?
2. What does it mean to be human?
3. How do we each live with greater joy, fulfillment, and peace?

While the goal of yoga may be interpreted differently, depending upon the underlying philosophy, for our purposes in the book it is understood to be a simultaneous path of liberation of the individual, *mokṣa*, and a path of union with all life and the Source of all beings. My hope is that the book's structure indeed brings you, the reader, to a place of greater inner freedom and unity.

Chapter 1

Subtle Bodies

Naturally, most people think of themselves as the container of their physical bodies. We may think of the skin as the outermost edge, holding together the complex structure of the various tissues and processes of the human body. Vedic teaching and Yoga, however, consider this a limitation arising from one of the many veils of illusion shrouding the true Self. One such limitation is the belief that we start and end with the container of the physical body. In Vedic teaching, beyond the physical body is a container of subtle energy, a *kośa* (pronounced kosha), that we refer to here as a "subtle body." Another limitation is not recognizing and not remembering the nature of the real Self. Part of this limitation is seeing the physical body as the real Self when it's the false self. Here, a distinction is made between the false or lower self and the real or true Self. (The small "s" and large "S" mark this distinction.)

In the journey toward inner liberation, the seeker is prodded to pull back the many obscurations that prevent them from seeing and living from their true Self. One path uses a framework such as the subtle bodies. Each subtle body has a specialized function, set of needs, and stage of mastery. Mastery occurs when all the lessons of that body are fully integrated and realized.

In a sense, there is an apparent paradox. On the one hand, the subtle bodies function like a cloak obscuring the real Self; on the other hand, they are a vehicle for the real Self to embody its unfolding fully. As a cloak, they provide the fuel that feeds the fire of learning and growth. For example, think about all the learning we are engaged in when we work through challenging emotions. We may "lose" ourselves when we so fully identify with an emotion that we forget who we truly are. As we'll discover, all emotions are primarily connected to the element of water. When water is not flowing, we can start to examine from where the stuckness originates.

As vehicles for exploring the inner dimensions of life, the subtle bodies provide a handrail of support in remembering who we truly are. The true Self, in simple terms, is energy. As energy, it is unlimited and entirely interconnected to the underlying and fundamental reality of all Consciousness. We may ask then, how does the Self as energy manifest?

We could think of it as an act of shrinking or condensing from something big to something small, a little bit like actor Rick Moranis' character in the movie *Honey, I Shrunk the Kids* (1989), albeit an overly simple analogy. The "something big" is the energy of an individual Self in non-physical terms. The "something small" is the individual Self that manifests in a material form, the physical body.

One of the first steps in the journey toward recognizing the true Self is for an individual to realize that they are more than the physical body itself. We come to recognize that the misidentification with the body as if it were the permanent self, is false. We further recognize that this reinforced idea of a permanent self, is in fact, temporary. The physical body eventually dies. The real Self is what is infinite and transcendent, living on beyond our concepts of time and space. The progression of this realization, of the transcendent Self, develops along the lines of the subtle bodies. One way we can think about suffering is a case of mistaken identity. Holding onto the idea that the false self is real and lasting, an individual remains caught in a web of illusion, like a hall of mirrors. True and lasting happiness resides within because the nature of the true Self is not limited nor separate. A separate self is one of the greatest illusions of them all. Everything is interconnected and interdependent. In the journey toward recognizing the true Self, each level of being is a boundary that is gradually integrated. Even though the subtle bodies inherently function as a boundary of separation, the seeker eventually realizes this boundary as necessary for the purpose of growth, experience, and evolution We could compare this to the realization that without darkness, we could not experience nor recognize that there is light.

The subtle bodies and the five elements are a framework that can help enlarge our understanding of ourselves. It can broaden our understanding of the relationships to each other, to Nature, and ultimately, the Source itself. One way to work within the framework involves locating areas of stagnation, blockages, or a lack of flow. As new insights, perspectives, and understanding become available, feelings of increased vitality and satisfaction may reflect the dissolving of the obstruction. This satisfaction further indicates that not only is more life force available, it is also flowing unobstructed. The greater the flow of life force and vitality, the closer we move toward the experiences of inner joy and peace.

Koshas

In the cosmological framework of an unfolding universe, one of the forces limiting or condensing individual experience is called Mayā. Usually ascribed a feminine pronoun, she is conceived of as the force or principle of obscuration. It is she who places limits in order for an individual experience to unfold. The energy of Mayā, the principal force of action and creativity, acting as an agent of Shakti, cloaks each individual within the subtle shrouds of illusion.

The five sheaths are:

1. Annamaya kośa – Physical body (composed of "food")
2. Prāṇamaya kośa – Life force (the link between the physical body and the mind)
3. Manomaya kośa – Mind (lower mind, desire and aversion)
4. Vijñānamaya kośa – Higher awareness (discernment, wisdom)
5. Ānandamaya kośa – Bliss (the transcendental Self)

Subtle Bodies

In 1875, Madame H.P. Blavatsky established the Theosophical Society (TS) based upon three objectives, one of which endeavors to discover the underlying fundamental truth of reality. With the society's founding, it laid the groundwork for a channel to transmit the ideas and experiences such as those explored by Tantric practitioners, from East to West. Annie Besant, an early disseminator of Theosophical teachings and views and a student of Madame Blavatsky, was a prolific writer, Sanskrit scholar, philosopher, and spiritual teacher. Dedicated to making the study of consciousness accessible to a broad audience of students, she sought to convey complex cosmic and philosophical subjects such that laypeople might easily undertake their study, thus expanding their thinking and spiritual development. One such areas of focus involved the subtle bodies. She believed that with the development of consciousness and fine tuning of the inner instruments of perception, a student could explore these subtle bodies for themselves.

Consciousness can assume different meanings depending on the context and the tradition in which it is being applied. The book uses the term to refer to a larger totality of an individual that is embodied, a level beyond what is usually thought of as the mind, personality/ego, and soul. Subtle bodies are non-physical containers formed of matter, which provide a structure as a vehicle for consciousness to experience itself and reality. I think of these subtle bodies as akin to nesting dolls. Each subtle body neatly fits "within" the other, roughly resembling the shape and outline of the physical body. Various practices, some of which are included in the book, help to develop and refine a practitioner's senses of perception. Through practice, it becomes possible to move one's awareness and focus from physical reality to non-physical reality, between the material and non-material realms of experience.

The model of the subtle bodies, as seen in Theosophical teachings, I believe makes a useful and insightful distinction with respect to the levels of mind. In many of the teachings found in Vedanta, the mind is conceived of as having a lower and higher function. The higher aspect is discriminative intelligence or *buddhi*. The lower mind is an aspect of both mental obscurations – *kleśas*, as well as emotions. By drawing out these two aspects of mind, it becomes more accessible for students to recognize the different states and functions. One of the most useful methods for exploring the mind is by employing the technique of categorization. In a sense, categorizing the mind as two distinct but connected states or levels, therefore, I believe, makes it easier to conceptualize. This distinction is important to note, I believe, as it helps to see the similarities between the subtle bodies and the koshas.

The subtle bodies as conceived of in Theosophy are:

1. Etheric Body – the physical body "doubled" in terms of subtle energy, also the body of vitality.
2. Astral/Emotional Body – the body of desire and emotions.
3. Mental Body – the body of beliefs, values, thoughts, and ideas.
4. Causal Body – the body of life purpose, the reincarnating self, and all the lifetimes of experience up to the present.
5. Buddhic Body – the body of unity consciousness, the transcendent Self, the blissful experience of oneness with all life.

Framework

Examining the relationships amongst the koshas, subtle bodies, and five elements illustrated in Table 1.1, it should be kept in mind that the nature of the subtle bodies is not a hierarchical structure. The layers interpenetrate, a little bit like nesting dolls. Individual consciousness itself is like a spatial point that is simultaneously apart from and connected to these interwoven layers. If we take the concept of the nesting dolls further, you could almost imagine that as each doll is removed from within the largest piece, they decrease in size and distance. This concept enables us to perceive them separately from the first doll to the last. The subtle bodies could similarly be imagined as extending outward, so to speak, from the physical body. As you move further out from the physical body, the more refined and less dense the energy field becomes. The more subtle the energy field, the harder it usually is to perceive. Awakening the inner instruments of perception and harnessing their latent potential, it becomes increasingly easier to perceive all the subtle bodies.

Table 1.1 – Relationships of the elements and subtle bodies

Kosha	Kosha (Yoga)	Subtle Body (Theosophy)	Five Elements
Food	Annamaya kośa	Dense Physical Body	Earth
Life Force	Prāṇamaya kośa	Physical double / Etheric Body	Earth
Emotions and Lower/ Sensory Mind	Manomaya kośa	Astral and Mental Body	Water (Astral) and Air Mental)
Intellect, discernment and wisdom	Vijñānamaya kośa	Causal Body	Fire
Transcendent Self and the bliss of that realization	Ānandamaya kośa	Buddhic Body	Ether/Space

Subtle Body exploratory practice

This short practice is a brief introduction to how we may begin exploring the energy field of the subtle vehicles of consciousness. Wherever you are right now, close your eyes. Start by paying attention to the contours of your physical body, where it meets the ground, and the surfaces that may be supporting it, such as a chair. Consider the areas where your skin has clothing touching the surface and where the skin is bare. Contemplate the entire surface area of skin encasing your physical body as the first edge, the first outermost boundary of your physical body. Next, concentrate on your breathing. As you feel the breath coming into your nose, consider that it is drawn in from a field of particles largely invisible to the naked eye. Imagine now, for a moment, that this field is lit up in some way. This field could be lit up with a color, or it could be somewhat colorless, like exhaling on a cold day and seeing your breath in the cold air. In your mind trace, this breath field like you did the contours of your physical body, except now the layer is only a few inches from the surface of your skin. If you are familiar with the concept of the human energy field as an aura, you can use that as your starting point. Now imagine that this breath field is replicated a few more times, the circle growing progressively larger and further away. You could mentally count outward as if each layer had a numerical value. "See" the layer closest to you, beginning with one and the layer furthest from you, as being five. Instead of or in addition using a numerical value, each layer can be perceived as having a different color, marking a clear distinction of each subtle body. As you extend your concentration out, notice how your awareness of yourself and your surroundings has shifted. Notice how great the effort to focus is as you reach inwardly to perceive these outer boundaries. Gradually, bring your attention back to your physical body once again, withdrawing your focus layer by layer. As you rest your attention in the body, take a few moments before opening your eyes to reorient yourself to your physical surroundings.

As a meditation practice, this is like basic training for developing the inner senses of perception as we learn to navigate these subtle realms of existence. With regular practice, it may become easier to perceive and recognize each of the bodies. To support this stage of practice, I recommend using a journal or piece of paper to write your experience and impressions. Keeping a meditation journal can help in the process of integrating what you learn during each meditation session.

Chapter 2

Cosmic Principles

The first answer that the Jîva shapes for himself to the great question, the first tentative solution of this overpowering doubt, is embodied in the view which is called the ârambha-vâda, the theory of a beginning, an origination, a creation of the world by an agency external to the questioner. From so-called fetish worship to highest deism and theism, all may be grouped under this first class of answer.

(Bhagaván Dás, *The Science of Peace*)

When I was in high school, part of the school curriculum included a weekly religious studies class. These classes were divided into two of the world's prominent religions, namely Christianity and Judaism. I was attending the class in Judaic studies. My young and inexperienced mind had an unanswered question, and the class presented a potentially ideal opportunity for answering it. So, I plucked up the courage and asked my then teacher if she could explain: *How could dinosaurs exist millions of years ago but the Jewish calendar was a little over 5000 years old?* I guess the answer was sufficiently satisfactory at that time. However, it did not completely erase a nagging feeling that there was something more to this story. This feeling led me to question the nature of reality, time, and the place of human beings within the universe.

Fast forward to early 2021, while writing this book, I happened to listen to a virtual online summit in which Deepak Chopra was amongst one of the speakers. The beginning of the presentation intrigued me. He suggested that his audience repeat the same Google web search he had done, namely, "What are the open questions in science?" I did just as he had suggested, corroborating what he'd said in his opening remarks; that 95% of the universe remains unknown. Some of these same questions in science are ones which I had asked myself as a young child. From the perspective of the statistical percentage, there is a great deal we do not yet know about the system of reality in which we find ourselves. Therefore, it makes sense that there remains a fundamental human drive to construct a framework that helps, in part, to answer some of the deepest questions we may, at one time or another, ask ourselves. In essence, the human endeavor seeks to understand the blueprint of the universe, of who we as human beings are, and, I would argue, how to live with peace and harmony.

Philosophy of the Tattvas

No truth is absolute. Each individual adopts a framework to construct and shape their worldview. What is true for one person may not be true for another. Each framework represents one perspective. Within the spectrum of all perspectives, for each individual, their perspective represents only one of the many perspectives possible. One framework this book draws upon is Indian philosophy, and more specifically, within the Tantric view of the Shaivite lineage of Kashmir. Four great sages from the northern region of India known as Kashmir developed this philosophy between the eighth to eleventh centuries AD. The philosophy and view that they elucidated came to be called the Doctrine of Recognition. An elegant and sophisticated explanation, this non-dual Tantric view manages to explain what, or rather, who has been forgotten. One way to think about this is a cast of characters, the two main ones being the real Self and the Source of all Being. The process of forgetting and remembering unfolds within this metaphysical framework in a sequence of thirty-six principles. Each of the thirty-six principles describes an aspect or property of matter, which themselves are called *tattvas*. Lacking an equivalent word within English, *tattva* means to express the quintessence of something, the very essential "that-ness" of a thing. Conceptually, these principles govern a particular aspect of reality and our experience. Consider the universal principle of gravity, which explains why we don't float on earth but do on the moon. This principle is universally true for every human being. In comparison, one of the tattvas governs the principle of the five senses.

This framework of the tattvas includes the five elements of nature, which themselves are related to and part of the five senses of perception. Although this is not the only spiritual framework based on the five elements, this particular perspective is one that has greater personal resonance for me over the others. The nagging feeling I'd had when I was younger, that there was more to reality than meets the eye, has found satisfaction within this cosmic framework.

It is possible to read the book, jumping ahead to the five elements directly, and skipping this next section entirely. However, for readers interested in a more detailed overview of the nature of this framework, this is detailed in the next section.

Cosmic Principles

There exists the idea that an Ultimate Reality upholds and permeates what we know to be our Universe. I refer to this ultimate reality simply as the Source, but it could be compared to or equated with similar names such as God, Logos, the Divine, Supreme Consciousness, Supreme Spirit, The Way, and so forth. The Tantric name given to describe this ultimate reality is *Parama Śiva*. Shiva represents the Source, and the prefix *Parama* emphasizes its placement in the cosmic order as supreme or ultimate.

It's natural to question why the Source created our universe with all of its particularities. Could we ever truly come to an answer that would be satisfactory? Unlikely, I would argue. I do, however, take the position that the Source began with a desire to know itself. With all of its omniscience, omnipresence, and omnipotence, the Source has the power to create. It has both the power and will to create, not just once, but unlimitedly. The Source exists before a tattva even comes into existence. From the power to create, we have a moment in which a universe unfolds and expands. This emerging unfolds aspects of the Source. Each phase is a step further out from the Source. Out of the oneness of the Source, it separates a portion of itself. This separation produces the first two principles contained within one seed, known as *Śiva* and *Śakti*. Shiva is the energy of life, life force, and vitality, and Shakti is the energy of form, creativity, and manifested reality. Comparatively, this would be thought of as Yin and Yang principles in Daoism. What appears as a duality is actually one of the root illusions. There is no duality but rather a relationship between the Source and the seed of separation, Shiva and Shakti. As with the concept of Yin and Yang, Shiva and Shakti both contain a portion of each other. And one of the simplest ways to conceive of this is that without darkness, we could not know and experience light, and vice versa. However, instead of duality, there is a triplicity which Annie Besant describes as three expressions of consciousness, namely *Will, Wisdom, and Activity* (Besant, A. p. 49). Wisdom (Shiva) is the expression of consciousness experiencing itself as "I am this." In the macro form, wisdom is the Source realizing itself, which is reflected in a micro form when an individual realizes the true Self. Activity (Shakti) is the expression of consciousness experiencing itself as "I am not this." In the macro form, activity is the Universal Self that creates and unfolds a Universe. This is reflected in a micro form as each individual having the power to create their own reality limitedly. Will (The Source) is the expression of consciousness experiencing itself as the relationship between the two others as the pure "I," the aspect of the Source that remains unchanged. In the macro form, Will is the Source withdrawing into the bliss of itself. In the micro

25

form, the individual abides in their true nature where self and not-self dissolve and merge into union with the Self. Trying to imagine what an exalted bliss state feels like, for the individual that has realized this in themselves, it is a deep realization of "the 'absolute rest and peace in one's own real self'" (Chatterji, J.C. p. 44). This is not to say that this is a one-time deal. Rather, I think we can have many experiences of inner realization that awaken in us a larger sense of Self, and this in turn may bring about a kind of inner bliss.

To more easily distinguish and thus contemplate the remaining phases of unfoldment, I suggest thinking of this in four stages. These are:

1. The first stage is where the world unfolds/manifests but is still hidden or veiled.
2. The second stage is where the unlimited powers of the Source are limited.
3. The third stage is where an individual spirit or soul begins to take form.
4. The fourth stage is manifestation of embodied physical form, expressions of the five elements.

The book's framework primarily focuses on the five elements but also includes a view into portions of the third stage.

Stage 1

In a world system, the first stage begins with manifestation. The Source unfolds a universe, first by separating a portion of itself. The Source imbues five states of consciousness with five characteristics of its omnipresence. As a distinction, these higher fivefold aspects are reflected later when the soul of an individual comes into being, in a lower or limited form. The fivefold aspects of the Universal process are:

1. *Cit* – The power to reveal the Self.
2. *Ānanda* – The power to realize the absolute bliss of the Self.
3. *Icchā* – The will to create.
4. *Jnāna* – The power to know.
5. *Kriyā* – The power to act and assume any form.

These fivefold characteristics are shared between the forces of Shiva and Shakti. Shiva contains the powers of self-revelation and the power to realize absolute bliss (numbers 1 and 2 above). Shakti, on the other hand, contains the will to create, the power to know, and the power to act and assume any form (numbers 3, 4, and 5 above).

In an individual, these forces are reflected as the capacity to realize the true Self, and the realization of the bliss of this true Self. It also means that there is the capacity to realize the knowledge and wisdom innate within the true Self and to bring this forward into conscious realization. An individual has the capacity to create their reality with the drive of their personal will, to act upon this will, and to bring it forward into any form in physical reality. This is what was meant earlier where the view in Theosophy points to a relationship between three primary expressions of consciousness, namely *Will*, *Wisdom*, and *Activity*.

Stage 2

This stage unfolds as soon as the impulse to take a form arises. All of the unlimited and transcendent aspects of the Source are now limited. This stage is known as *Maya*, a Sanskrit term roughly meaning "illusion." Referred to in the feminine form, Maya symbolizes the force of obscuration and limitation. As she stretches her power of obscuration, she wraps herself like a cloak around the manifested world, simultaneously enfolding herself within it. The veil she shrouds around the world to restrain the Source's unlimited powers is by way of five special coverings:

1. Time (*Kāla*) – Individuals experience a past, present, and future instead of the reality of all time as being simultaneous. Time, including the concept of eternity, is an idea, not a real reality. Through inner realization, an individual experiences the "now."

2. Knowing (*Vidyā*) – The experience of knowing everything is limited. This all-knowing includes knowledge of the true Self. An individual must eventually realize that all reality is a projection of the Self, including the feeling of separation and duality.

3. Desire (*Rāga*) – An individual feels a sense of lacking something; the search to fulfill that lack leads to desire, wanting something or someone, and or not wanting something or someone. In the pursuit to fulfill this perceived "lack of something," the result is a feeling of never fully being satisfied. An individual must realize the real message behind the yearning, which is to be in union with all things and all beings.

4. Authorship (*Kalā*) – Although each individual has the power to create their reality, they are limited in their ability to create (*kriyā*) what they want, whenever they wish or think of what they want. These limitations ensure an alignment with the Divine Will.

5. Determinism (*Niyati*) – Every individual's growth conditions are bound by the law of *karma*, essentially cause and effect, which limits personal, or individual will. In a system based on the principles of learning and growth, reality creation is sufficiently slowed down such that individuals may learn from the consequences of their intentions and actions.

Stage 3

In this stage, an individual spirit/soul begins to take form as a single unit, a unit of unique consciousness. To conceptualize this more easily, we can think of this as having two parts, namely Part A and Part B. The components making up an individual unit of consciousness is Part A. From the many billions of souls on the planet, how a unique spirit/soul expresses itself is Part B.

Part A

In this part, we have the principle of the subject-object relationship. Subject (*Purusha*) and object (*Prakriti*) exist simultaneously. Think of this as a single coin with two sides. One side represents the observer or witness (subject); the other represents the observed or participant (object). When beginning meditators learn the first foundation of mindfulness, which is observing the breath, the practice reflects the ability a person has to observe their breath while they are at the same, the breath itself. The act of breathing is participatory, whereas the act of watching is witnessing.

Subject (*Purusha*) and object (*Prakriti*) echo earlier stages of manifestation. The echo exists as one side has the experience of, *I am this/that*, whereas the other has the experience of *I am not this/that*. As a meditator refines their attention and awareness skills, they eventually develop the ability to recognize these two principles clearly. The next stage of meditation opens to the subject-object experience falling away. Now, a meditator can flow their attention in a merged state of concentration. We now see, facilitated through meditation, a gradual realization that duality is an idea and not a reality. In other words, our thoughts and ideas are projected onto the screen of the physical world which itself is a composite of the materials of matter.

Part B

When we think of our day-to-day reality, we are relating to the unseen forces that created it. This creation is Prakriti (object), which manifests reality through three modes called *gunas*. A guna is an aspect of, or property of, matter (matter being the substance of existence). These three modes initially exist in a state of equilibrium. When this equilibrium is disturbed, to create a unique individual spirit or soul, the three modes manifest in various permutations. The three modes are:

1. Sattva – rhythm, vibration, and harmony
2. Rajas – mobility and action
3. Tamas – inertia, calm, and the power of resistance

I have opted to use the less well-known definitions of the gunas as translated by Annie Besant. I feel they offer a more direct experience of the energy that the gunas themselves express throughout our cosmic universe.

At this stage, as the three gunas move out of equilibrium, several permutations can be combined, which, according to Besant, produce a *"septenate"* (Besant, A. pp. 75–77). These divisions of seven groups reflect a higher or lower expression of each of the gunas. So, for example, and this is purely illustrative, one permutation might be 20% sattva, 60% rajas, and 20% tamas. What is important to note with these permutations is the variety that is created, giving rise to different combinations and expressions in each individual soul and the unique paths for learning and growth. It can also offer a different perspective of how or why there might be an imbalance in an individual, or some challenge a person may be having difficulty with overcoming. Whether we know it or not, we're always striving for balance. Think of how it feels when we are experiencing good health and easeful living versus a stressful day and some sort of physical distress.

Systems like Ayurveda and Hatha yoga utilize the gunas and the five elements as a way of looking at the essential constitution of a person which is called a dosha. If there is an imbalance, it is often traced back to the interaction of the elements and the gunas. And similarly, working with the elements and the gunas is a way of maintaining balance. Food and herbs can also be described according to their perceived elemental combinations. Something hot and spicy like habanero chilis could be described as being rajasic, because of its ability to generate heat in the body. This heat will typically lead to sweating, whether it's a light perspiration or beads dripping down the back of a shirt. Conversely, something sweet and cooling like a watermelon could be described as sattvic, with its ability to cool the body and sweeten the mind. This view is interesting in two ways. First, we can relate to Part A when a unique soul comes into being. There may indeed exist many similarities, but there are just enough parameters to create the conditions of unique expression. Second, one task for each individual in their path back to the Source is to bring the gunas back into equilibrium. We could imagine this as feeling something like "calm awareness, moving passion and dulling stupefaction" being in an ideal state of equilibrium once again (Chatterji, J.C. p. 50–51).

In the last stages of manifestation, the five elements themselves are affected by how the modes impose their qualities onto matter. As we keep in mind the qualities of the gunas, our efforts to restore equilibrium may be better informed and more effective. This understanding is additive – the more we can understand this for ourselves, the better equipped we are to understand this in others. One way we can think of working with the energy of the gunas is to think of the actions that they each represent as a starting point for establishing or reestablishing harmony and flow in the form of a question:

1. Sattva – If we think of the energy of harmony as right knowledge, from which self-insight and compassion arise, we might ask the question: *Am I acting in service of the greater good of all, including myself?* A higher perspective

31

and greater understanding enable us to see what the appropriate next step or set of steps are, within the rubric of non-harm.

2. Rajas – If we think of the energy of mobility as right action, from which flow-based living arises, we might ask the question: *Am I in alignment with a call to act from the Soul?* Living in flow is not only possible; it is joyful, particularly as we operate from a call to act from our highest selves.

3. Tamas – If we think of the energy of stability as right desire, from which responsiveness to growth arises, we might ask the question: *Are my actions in alignment with my dharma and the dharma of the Universe?* The more we are open to change, with a willingness to learn and grow, the easier it becomes to align personal intentions with universal intentions. Conversely, resistance to change or insisting your way over others is a bit like trying to swim upstream. Resistance diminishes the available flow of life force and instead, there is less flow which naturally leads to feeling stuck.

An important skill we will be working with throughout the book in an effort to restore and maintain equilibrium begins with inquiry. From a position of curiosity and a desire to know more, we are lifted to see things from a higher perspective where it becomes possible to examine the energy these forces exert in all spheres of life.

Stage 4

Finally, a soul comes into form, weaving together a higher intellect, mind, personality-ego, and a physical and subtle body formed of the five elements. As the soul becomes embodied in physical form, it takes on a unique combination of the properties of matter. The unique combinations create variety and differentiation that is then expressed into material form.

The unfolding of differentiation from subtle space to material earth is expressed through five subtle elements (tanmātras), five sense organs (panca jñānendriya), five motor organs of action of the physical body (panca karmmendriya), and five great elements as the dense forms of material matter (panca mahabhutas).

Table 2.1. Expression of the five elements

Space/Ether (Ākāśa)	Fire (Agni)	Air (Vāyu)	Water (Ap)	Earth (Prthvī)
Sound (Shabda)	Sight (Rūpa)	Touch (Sparsha)	Taste (Rasa)	Smell (Gandha)
Ear/Sound (Auditory)	Eye/Vision (Sight)	Hand/ Tactile (Touch)	Tongue (Taste)	Smell/ Nose (Olfaction)
Expression/ Speech (Mouth)	Locomotion (Feet)	Manipulation of physical environment (Hand)	Emission and Procreation (Urino Genital)	Digestion and Elimination (Anus)
Communication and self-expression becoming physical form	Perception and movement	Movement of thought	Flow and movement	Solidity and stability

Even though the unlimited Self is cloaked and "hidden" from itself, it retains its capacity to be self-aware. Self-awareness expresses itself in the subject-object relationship. Consciousness can experience itself as both the witness and the participant. Although Consciousness retains the capacity of self-awareness, this is forgotten, hidden behind the functions of the ego-personality, the lower mind, and the various sensory potentials. With each level of differentiation, from the physical body to the mind, these become vehicles that facilitate a returning journey for the unlimited Self to re-remember itself. This becomes a framework then for Self-realization, a path for transcending from the realm of the material to the subtle and from illusion to truth. This marks the quest, a spiritual journey that each individual takes inward toward the true Self and ultimately, to the Source of all beings.

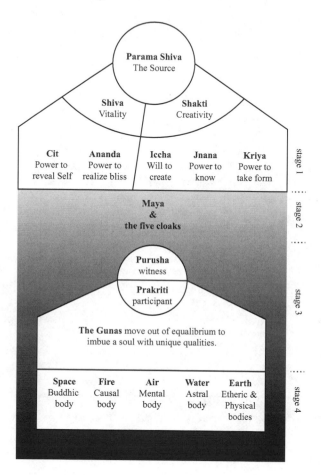

Chapter 3

The Five Elements

If we examine the mechanism by which reality is experienced, we see that it is largely one of representing, using, and interpreting through the means of symbols. This may be easier to conceptualize when the symbols have a physical form. A painting, for instance, expresses the thoughts, feelings, and values of the artist. Clothing represents cultural and personal identity. Language is a vehicle of communication conveying needs, ideas, meaning, and intention by converting the energy of an idea or thought into a symbol, the symbol being the spoken words themselves.

The models of human experience, and our understanding of them, are themselves evolving. One of the ways we can observe the evolution of symbols is in language. The meaning of a word or phrase today may differ greatly in its meaning from its use a hundred years ago. I believe that any framework we use is simply a vehicle for navigating and evolving along the journey of learning of growth. As my work grew in teaching and healing others, I became especially interested in synthesizing a framework that would benefit others to expand their own spiritual self-development. The evolution of this interest grew into working with the five elements. Whether or not we are consciously aware of them, the five elements of earth, water, air, fire, and space surround us all the time. A meta-view of the elements provides, I believe, an ideal template for exploring and unfolding the subtle levels of being. As important, I believe it also provides a way forward to restore our relationship with Nature. One of the principles underlying our universe is *interdependence*. Suffering, as well as freedom from suffering, does not happen in a vacuum. It is a multi-sensory, multi-dimensional experience.

I have several houseplants, some of which have been in my care for more than ten years. If I neglect the care they need – adequate light sources, fresh air, replenishment of nutrients, water – they respond by wilting, dropping their leaves, possibly even death. Self-care is similar in that when we fail to nourish the body, mind, and spirit properly, the symptoms are not dissimilar to the wilting house plant.

The hubris of disconnection that largely severed the relationship in which human beings recognized, celebrated, and cherished the interdependence with Nature is facing a reckoning as alarm bells sound on climate change. While the book's subject does not specifically focus on climate change, we cannot ignore our relationship to the environment in the pursuit of spiritual growth. For instance, forest bathing has become a recent buzzword, encouraging people especially isolated from nature, to get outside and immerse themselves within the cocoon of peace and tranquility that can be found in the woods. However, without forests, there can be no forest bathing. Spiritual practices that invite us to use nature for inner exploration and rejuvenation need a deeper recognition of the environment's vital role. Otherwise, it becomes another form of simply taking without reciprocity.

On an individual level, full-spectrum change and healing are often incomplete when the higher and more subtle levels of being are not acknowledged and integrated. Increasingly, there is greater recognition and acceptance of the body-mind-emotion-spirit connection in various modalities. Somatic therapies, for instance, see a link between the thoughts and feelings of a past trauma that later becomes stored in the physical body. Modern civilization often refers to the stress of living and working in big cities. Stress is the umbrella term for a variety of thoughts and feelings as a reaction to the pushes and pulls of daily living in the often fast-paced life of these larger and more condensed cities. The symptoms of stress are varied, such as hypertension, digestive issues, headaches, sleep disturbances, exhaustion, and more. As we'll see later in the book, it's possible to examine all areas of our lives, including our relationships with others, from the perspective of the elements and whether or not they are in or out of balance.

Foundation

The central principle of the framework is balance and there are four components to this:

1. Recognizing imbalances
2. Restoring balance
3. Maintaining balance
4. Uniting all the elements

As you work through the practices, it should be borne in mind that although you may restore balance to one or more of the elements today, they may be out of balance once again a month later. This is because one of the principles of reality is the nature of impermanence. Life is always changing; there is a constant ebb and flow. The practices in the book are designed to support you through this ever-changing flow of living.

A second principle of the framework is needs. Each level of being has a specific set of needs, and this is universal to all human experience. There are four components:

1. Through recognition and subsequent fulfillment of the needs particular to each level of being, optimal functioning is supported.
2. Because the levels are interwoven, fulfillment of needs at one level has a corresponding impact on one or more of the other levels.

3. As needs are met, more life force becomes available, which corresponds with a rising feeling of satisfaction.

4. Joy is then the natural result, arising out of the present moment.

When one or more needs is satisfied, it fulfills one of the most universal of all human desires:

1. the need to be seen
2. the need to be heard
3. the need to be understood

When we see that what connects us is greater than what seems to divide us, the possibility to meet one another with empathy and compassion expands. This can be summed up in one word – harmony. And it touches three areas – harmony in oneself, harmony with others, and harmony with Nature.

As you investigate each of the elements, keep in mind that they are not like silos, standing alone and separate. The elements and the subtle bodies are interrelated, interwoven, and interpenetrating. This comes together more fully in the section that deals specifically with balancing elements.

Chapter 4

Earth

Our journey begins with earth, the first element and the foundation upon which our human bodies stand. The essence of the earth element is the principle of form-building. Any experience an individual intends to bring into material reality begins with an idea, which may eventually manifest itself into physical form. Form building is represented in the physical body as the instrument of action on the physical plane. The body is simultaneously the container for the unlimited Self and the vehicle through which the Self experiences learning and growth in material reality. One of the lessons of the earth element is the degree to which we are able to ground our experiences in physical reality. This means becoming fluent in translating the energy of ideas and lessons – the non-visible and non-material, into an embodied lived experience.

Think of a potter who will form an idea in their mind of something they wish to create, such as a bowl. The bowl will have a purpose – it could be a cereal bowl, for instance, with certain dimensions and an overall shape. With a good clear image of the bowl, the potter gets to work shaping a lump of clay. The potter needs to be able to develop their idea of a bowl, aligning the concept with their intention – a vessel for breakfast consumption, for example, and then follow through step by step, action by action, for it to materialize. Whether baking a loaf of bread, writing a thesis, composing a symphony, or moving cities, all of these endeavors are the creative impulse of life shining forth.

The impulse to create is intertwined at all levels of life, within each of us and around us. What we call "life force" is more than the breath and air we take in that sustains our life. As the creative principle, at a micro-level, it is the energy and vitality that pulsates in every cell in the body; at a macro-level, it is the pulsation of life flowing through the very heart of the Universe itself. The fullness of our life force is always available to us, but its flow increases or decreases depending on the degree to which that flow is restricted or not. As with the potter who needs to center the clay lest it resists being shaped, individuals also need to be centered to more easily channel the flow of life. When life force is restricted or seemingly depleted, usually the health and vitality of the physical body is affected. A greater influx of life force flowing through the body increases the feeling of well-being, with more reserves available to pursue activities and actions on the physical plane. Less life force means there is less exuberance, motivation, and plain old "oomph"!

In addition to being the creative impulse and life force, the subtle energy field surrounding the physical body – the etheric body, is also a conduit. In a sense, the etheric body is a channel for converting and relaying impressions, vibrations, and energy arising from the higher subtle bodies and the external environment into forms that can be taken up in the physical body. In other words, it is a link between the body and the mind. We can influence this energy field when using the insight and wisdom of the mind, thereby placing our conscious awareness upon the impressions of thoughts, sensations, and feelings. As we become more sensitive to and present with this bi-directional flow of information between the body and mind, we cultivate the ability to better direct our focus and actions.

We become more effective at grounding thoughts and ideas when the basic needs of embodied physical consciousness are met. More space is available for a greater flow and influx of life force into the body by meeting and satisfying these needs.

The needs of the body are examined in five categories: food, sanctuary, rest, movement, and presence.

Food

While it may be clichéd to say, the body is indeed a temple. It is not uncommon not only to **not** think about the body but to treat it as nothing more than a machine. And it can go in the extreme opposite direction by valuing the body only materialistically. Overstating the obvious bears repeating – consciousness would not be able to live, learn, and grow in physical reality without a body. Food, therefore, symbolizes satisfaction in material and non-material terms.

One of the body's most basic needs is derived from a wholesome diet that is as natural and as unprocessed as possible. As with most things in life, moderation is the key. Wholesome foods provide most of the nutrients and calories the body needs to maintain optimal function. And when the body is healthy and has a lot of energy, it's possible to pursue other daily activities with ease and enjoyment, like walking up a flight of stairs or hiking three miles.

In non-material terms, food is the connection between the digestion of experiences – how we felt or thought about something. Consider for a moment how it feels to eat, for instance, lunch under the shade of a tree on a sunny day. And then compare that feeling to eating the same meal inside a busy food court inside a shopping mall. The inward relationship to those experiences will be different – enjoyment and satisfaction will vary. When there is a feeling of greater pleasure and satisfaction, there is more life force available. Remember, there is a direct relationship between levels of satisfaction and life force.

Taking this concept deeper, we can think of the connection between food and the willingness to try new cuisines or new flavors. This willingness is symbolized as the *variety of experiences*. Staying open to new experiences opens up more possibilities than can be imagined by the mind alone. In other words, a willingness to investigate foods not ordinarily part of one's daily diet expands consciousness and develops greater flexibility of mind.

Mindfulness of eating goes beyond what we consume in support of physical health and well-being. Mindfulness of eating needs to include the relationship to Nature's cyclic rhythms and one's impact on the Earth. By considering how we get our food and from where, we establish one of the core principles of balancing all the elements: harmony. As the world grapples with climate change, each step in the food chain has implications on our individual and collective footprint.

The ideal, when satisfying a personal need, is finding the balance between self-care and care of others, including the earth itself.

Sanctuary

Everyone needs a place where they feel safe, protected, and at peace. Suppose we are fortunate enough to have a home with all the essentials covered – clean running water, consistent electricity, heating/cooling, a place to sleep and eat, more possibilities open to establishing the home to feel like a sanctuary. A home, in general, can aspire to create a space that feels tranquil, calm, peaceful. Still, it may be that smaller areas are dedicated to this given the variety of living situations (living alone versus with roommates or a family, etc.) that abound. It may be possible to identify a corner or room as a special space for meditation and contemplation. The starting point here is to create a clean, ordered, organized space and free of excessive clutter.

Some readers may be familiar with organizing expert Marie Kondo. Her philosophy is applicable here, in which individuals ask inwardly if the objects in the home "spark joy." Essentially, it is an invitation to consider whether *things* in the home are meaningful and have an additive or reductive effect. Sanctuary is finding an ideal balance between austerity and overconsumption so that everything in the space contributes to the intention.

Rest

We are habituated to thinking that a nightly ritual of eight hours of sleep is primarily when the body rests, recharges, and renews itself. Sleep is certainly important but, there are other routines and practices to consider. The key to remember is that with appropriate rest, more energy becomes available to maintain focus, concentration and, ultimately, be fully present. As a general practice, a first step recognizes the signals from the body when energy reserves start to wane. A shortlist for jump-starting the tank, so to speak, can include closing your eyes for five or ten minutes and sitting quietly. A "power nap" for twenty minutes, whether mid-morning or mid-afternoon, can also be a great recharge. There are practices such as yoga nidra and restorative yoga, which teach, amongst other things, how to slow down and allow the body to receive support to relax and recharge. Another form of rejuvenation and rest is sitting outside. Imagine a park bench beneath the shade of a tree, listening to the surrounding sounds, enjoying the time to sit and be. If we listen to Nature, beneath the hum of activity, the sounds of birds chirping or the wind blowing, it is actually very quiet. By immersing ourselves in Nature, we instinctively return to the same underlying inner quiet within ourselves. Within this quiet is the well-spring of life force. It can sound a bit like an oxymoron – that to connect, we need to disconnect. Pressure builds up in the body from the various pushes and pulls of daily life. It's no wonder that the energy of 5 p.m. traffic is so intense – people leaving work at the end of a busy day are desperate to get home to rest. Restorative activities and rest are the release valve for the pressure build-up. In general, people are more present and calm when they've had appropriate rest.

Movement

Essential to the maintenance of optimal health and well-being of the body are movement and exercise. Activities that promote light sweating, oxygenation of the blood, expanding the lungs and the heart, and so on are all important for maintaining health. A shortlist includes but is not limited to walking, swimming, hiking, biking, running, postural yoga, tai chi, Pilates, and more. As an added bonus, exercising and moving outside connects and reconnects us with Nature, which, as we've already noted, is a source of recharge and renewal.

Presence

Stress, tension, worry – these are only a few of the emotions that can affect ways in which the body becomes wound up in tightness, constriction, and discomfort. Consider the tortoise for a moment, with its hard protective shell into which it can withdraw under duress or extend out from when safe. In a similar sense, consciousness withdraws itself from the body under pressure and needs to be welcomed back into the body. One way for consciousness to become re-embodied is facilitated through various modalities of healing bodywork and energy work. Some examples include the Alexander Technique, Rolfing, Chiropractics, Reiki, Acupuncture, and Thai Massage. Other modalities that assist the re-grounding of consciousness in the body involve working with animals, such as equine-assisted therapy and canine-assisted therapy. Showing up and staying present in the moment is infinitely greater once we are able to be grounded and fully embodied. Being fully present is an ideal to strive for, which may take months, years, or a lifetime to live from day to day. Small moments of effort become larger moments over time. A good way to practice this can be likened to walking – take one step at a time, one foot in front of the next.

Summary – Skillful Action

As with all the elements, we develop familiarity with them over time, especially with the ones with which we are less comfortable. More proficiency develops the more familiar we become with each element. We become more capable and effective at creating our reality on the physical plane. There is a feeling of accomplishment and satisfaction that arises and an embodied skill of the form building principle itself. The true Self is able to and is supported in fully expressing itself in all its radiant beauty.

Earth element practice – Grounding meditation

This practice is intended to put us in touch with the qualities of stability and groundedness of the earth element, feeling the sensations through the body, which is facilitated with direct contact with the ground. Direct contact reminds us of our spiritual, non-material Self's connection to our material Self in the body. If possible, try the practice outside where it's possible to be in touch with Nature, such as a park or garden. Of course, the practice can be done inside where access to such outside space is not available. The instructions provided for this meditation assume a standing position. However, the practice is perfectly suitable for sitting or lying down. If standing and where balance is difficult with closed eyes, leaning against a wall is a suitable addition to the practice.

To begin, locate a place that is relatively quiet and free of distraction. Come into a comfortable standing position, placing the feet about shoulder-width apart and letting the arms hang loosely along the sides of the body. Look straight ahead for a moment, positioning the head pointing neither downward nor upward but rather in a relatively neutral and open position. Before closing the eyes, imagine the feet sinking into the ground as if making an indentation in the ground. Feel as though this creates a sensation of stabilizing your position, like roots anchoring a tree in its place. Gradually closing the eyes, bring your focus inward. Using the inner visual sense perception, bring your inner gaze to where the body meets the ground, the feet. Notice the subtly shifting of body weight, a gentle and slight sway, like a tree moving gently in a light breeze. Feel that both feet hold the weight of the body equally. Expand the sensation of stability and connection to the ground upward and outward, growing up through the legs toward the crown of the head, outward to just a few inches beyond the outermost edge of the physical body. Imagine drawing up from the Earth the energies of growth, vitality, stability, and support as you inhale. As you exhale, imagine radiating these energies upward and outward, throughout the whole physical body and into the personal energy field boundary that is a few inches from the skin's surface. It can be helpful to visualize not only the qualities of the energy but also the color, which for the earth element is green. When we think of trees in their full stature and glory, the greenery of the leaves displays all of their full vibrancy and aliveness. Imagine the sensation of vibrant aliveness pulsing throughout the physical and energetic body. To bring the practice to a close, take a moment to hold a feeling of deep heartfelt gratitude in the mind. Feel a gentle smile softening across the face and the heart rising and opening like a blooming flower on a warm spring day. Open the eyes gradually, slowly returning to the outer surroundings before continuing with the day.

Going deeper

Consider for a moment that all the elements are present in the physical body. The body is always striving for balance as a consciousness of its own. We balance the elements through the food we eat, the information we consume, and how we move, such as exercise. The postural practice of yoga, with its focus on breath and mindfulness, is one of the many ways we can work with the five elements within ourselves. To illustrate this in practice, we could think about developing a movement session based upon three components:

1. Energetic focus
2. Physical focus
3. Practice focus

Energetic focus directs attention to either one element specifically or some combination of the elements. Physical focus directs attention to what we want the body to do, such as lengthening versus contracting. With practice focus, we direct attention to the actual poses that support guiding the energetic focus. By thinking of all three, it may be possible to direct the flow of energy, attention, and awareness in a way that enlivens the element not only in the moment but also within ourselves. Therefore, the template can be applied creatively, whether you are practicing for yourself or teaching it to others in an individual or group session.

As with the beginning of any postural yoga practice, there should be a period where the muscles are adequately warmed up and prepared, particularly for more physically demanding poses. Although actual sample practices have not specifically been outlined, a general familiarity and experience with the practice of yoga poses have been assumed.

Earth Element

Energetic focus:
- groundedness
- vitality and well-being of the body
- touching the energetic center of the earth.

Physical focus:

- stability, firmness & strength in the legs
- equal balance when standing on both feet, in body & mind
- standing in the center of your being
- moving with steadiness

Practice focus:

- standing poses, emphasizing grounding through the legs and feet such as:
- Mountain Pose (*Tadasana*)
- Equal Standing Pose (*Samasthitih*)
- Triangle Pose (*Trikonasana*)
- Tree Pose (*Vrksasana*)

Water Element

Energetic focus:

- flow
- fluidity
- ease and grace

Physical focus:

- gentle movements that lengthen out through the extremities, a feeling of reaching up and out through the arms and hands
- graceful transitions between movements emphasizing continuity and connection between poses
- movements connected to one another suggestive of flowing water

Practice focus:

- movements along the spine that shift the body forward, backward, side-to-side, and in rotation such as:
- Seated or kneeling cat/cow pose (*Marjariasana/Bitilasana*)

- Revolved side angle pose (*Parivrtta Parsvakonasana*)
- Bridge pose (*Setu Bandhāsana*)
- Bow pose (Dhanurasana)

Air Element

Energetic focus:
- perspective
- seeing the world including oneself through new eyes and new possibilities
- trying new things

Physical focus:
- movements that instill a feeling of lightness in the body, such as:
- using various props such as blankets or bolsters that provide support and open one to the feeling of being lifted up and or held
- using the wall as a practice tool with the perspective of exploring the body relative to an unmoving object

Practice focus:
- Supported reclining chest opening pose (*Supta Matsyasana*)
- Supported Child's pose (*Balasana*)
- Inverted leg position or "Legs up the wall" pose (*Viparita Karani*)
- Bridge pose at the wall (*Setu Bandhāsana*)

Fire Element

Energetic focus:
- building heat
- stimulating enthusiasm
- playfulness

Physical focus:

- stimulating movements that are rhythmic
- mobilizing and freeing the joints
- warming up the body through sequential, repetitive movements
- using the power of heat to transform the body and the mind
- burning up what is not needed as fuel for the body and light for the mind

Practice focus:

- cultivating endurance and stamina:
- The Sun Salutation sequence (*Surya Namaskar*)
- Half Moon Pose (*Ardha Chandrasana*)
- Chair pose (*Utkatasana*)
- Side Plank pose (*Vasisthasana*)

Space Element

There are two primary vehicles for exploring the element of space in the body. The first involves making conscious the effort to pause between each movement or series of movements and notice the "gap" between them. This gap can be likened to the natural pause that exists between each inhale and exhale. It's a moment that is there; it exists; we need only turn our attention to it and recognize it, welcome it, and bathe in it. The second involves the receptive quiet that is received when a physical movement practice is concluded. The conclusion of the practice is not simply a moment to rest or catch one's breath. It's an invitation for consciousness to become aware of itself, aware of the body and the ways the body's own consciousness is integrating various pushes and pulls. Typically, this may be more comfortable to explore lying down on one's back, but it could be equally enlightening sitting with or without support for the back, such as from a wall or a chair. This practice of becoming aware of the space between something could be expanded and explored outside of physical movement practice. Some ideas to explore could include the end of a meal before moving on to the next activity or task, like washing the dishes and sitting for a few moments before driving off to the next destination at the end of a long hike. Instead of trying to fill a silent pause during a conversation, let the space expand, taking in the exchange of words and energy between one another. Lean into the element of space instead of away from it.

Chapter 5

Water

Water is made up of three atoms: one oxygen molecule and two hydrogens molecules. This makeup gives water some special properties – water can be both liquid and solid, transforming the flowing state such as a lake to frozen ice. If you fill a bucket with water, you may notice that carrying water is actually quite heavy. Water holds varying degrees of temperature, a spectrum ranging from high heat to very cold. It can also generate immense momentum and force – compare a gushing waterfall to a gentle stream or the trickle of a babbling brook. Water is a powerful and essential element for the maintenance and sustenance of all life.

For all of its various properties, water is the messenger of flow. And as the sustainer of life, it nourishes the flow of life force, vitality, energy, and growth. Emotions are intimately connected with this element. Whatever feeling arises, it signals how life force is flowing, either increasing or decreasing in greater or lesser satisfaction rates. In language, metaphors express this relationship between the water element and our emotions – *to cry a river, their eyes welled with tears, they gushed with pride, as furious as a rainstorm*. Emotions, their purpose, and their value are often misunderstood. A river, once graceful and free-flowing, is obstructed when a large dam wall is constructed. Now the river can't flow freely anymore. Over time, pressure continues to build because the river wishes to be free. The built-up pressure eventually generates enough force to break the dam wall, causing flooding as it rushes toward freedom. Emotions are analogous to this. If they are pent up with no opportunity to be appropriately channeled or expressed, they eventually build up until they either spillover or burst. Learning to channel emotions and ride its waves is one of the water element lessons, a skill developed in meditation practices aimed toward cultivating equanimity.

Contrary to popular belief, there is a misperception that, in the pursuit of cultivating equanimity, an individual would somehow need *not* have emotions. This misperception also includes the idea that equanimity is detachment, especially in the domain of loving relationships. In the Yoga Sūtras of Patanjali, it is said that "yoga is the cessation of the modifications of the mind." In broad terms, this means that for a practitioner of Yoga (yogin [male] or yoginī [female]) to experience liberation and union, they would need to develop the ability to remain steady, calm, and tranquil without being disturbed by emotions as they arise. The practitioner can observe the emotions (which are the modifications), be present with them, understand them, but is not pulled into their ups and downs such that they lose their tranquil calmness. The skills for cultivating this kind of tranquil state of consciousness are developed as a twofold process. The first step in the process involves working with the water element to understand what emotions are and how to maintain a sense of balance when they arise. The second stage works with the air element, which we cover specifically under that heading. Charles calls this state "joyful clarity," which is living from and maintaining a state of tranquil consciousness. In the section on practices, we offer some methods that are a beginning point for establishing oneself in this joyful clarity.

The water element not only governs emotions. It also controls how we interpret the flow of experience(s). Whereas earth is about action, water is about movement. Any idea that we want to bring into physical reality needs to be able to flow without obstruction. That doesn't mean that there won't be some obstacles; rather, it's about recognizing the forces providing the clearest path possible for that idea to manifest. As an analogy, we can think about any idea or project starting like a water droplet. The water droplet, say from a rain cloud, looks for a suitable carrier. It could be a river; it could be a stream; it could be an ocean. Let's say that the water droplet chooses a small brook minding its own business in a quiet woodland forest. As the water droplet joins with the brook, it begins to gather momentum. It's hardly noticeable since the brook is just barely a trickle. But, as the brook travels along its path, it joins up with a large creek that's quite vibrant. Now, our tiny water droplet has some real momentum behind it. As the creek flows, rushing over and around the rocks, it suddenly comes to an abrupt stop. A family of beavers has constructed their dam, blocking the flow of the creek. Our water droplet is stuck, albeit temporarily. Eventually, the water droplet squeezes through the beavers' obstacle course, meeting upstream with a river. As it joins the river, momentum gathers once again until finally, the water droplet enters its planned destination – a large lake. It will stay here for some time until it's ready to be pulled back up into the clouds, this time for a journey to an ocean.

Like our tiny water droplet, a project or some area of Self-expression may have difficulty finding an appropriate balance of flow and momentum. Swamps are areas saturated with water, where water doesn't move very much. As an imbalance, too much water can feel as though a person is swamped – possibly due to a lack of organization or time management skills, perhaps due to taking on more than can be adequately managed. An imbalance of too much water that is stagnant, like the swamp, can also feel as though it's difficult to gather yourself together. Not only is the water a little stuck and stagnant, but it's also quite spread out. Each person's energy can be spread out everywhere – a kitchen sink full of dishes that have piled up over three days; or stacks upon stacks of paperwork hiding the fact that there is actually a desk beneath it all! There's also the contrast between an overbooked doctor whose calendar is swamped with back-to-back appointments versus the self-employed gig worker traveling all over the place and spread too thin. A balanced water element reflects an ability to gather momentum like a wave, ride the wave, and eventually pour itself out into manifest reality instead of falling off the wave to be pulled under a churning undercurrent.

Fluidity with the water element is supported by its own set of core needs, which facilitate the flow of life force moving easily or overcoming any obstacles along the way.

Emotional support

An essential component of a balanced water element is the need for emotional support. Emotions tell a story, and they facilitate a way for us to express how we feel about ourselves, each other, and the world around us. Emotions connect us with our beliefs and values, where they may act as a spokesperson for how we might wish to express those worldviews. Relationships and environments that support the expression of feelings and emotions are critical if there is to be a feeling of sufficient safety for a person(s) to open up. The expression and sharing of emotions are twofold. There is the willingness to be vulnerable in opening up and sharing, and second, there is the safety created when the vulnerability is welcomed and respected. One of the ways a relationship is sustained and deepened is a willingness to be open, be vulnerable, and share a heart-to-heart connection. This is true whether the relationship is with a best friend, a life partner, a colleague – a heart-to-heart connection can be shared even with a stranger. Areas in life where it's not possible nor wise to be open and vulnerable are counterbalanced by spending time with people with whom a close bond is shared. Sometimes, emotional support comes in the form of a deeply held knowing gaze, a long hug, or placing a hand on the person's shoulder. And it's important to remember to harness the power of your own agency to ask for what you need. Asking for a hug or a friend to sit quietly with you opens the heart and the space for connection.

Emotional fluency

As with learning a new language, emotions are their own unique vocabulary. Fluency with emotions involves learning the range of possible emotions, their value when they show up, and how to navigate working with them to ensure that life force continues to flow freely. A balance is cultivated when learning to discern how to appropriately express and channel emotions, knowing when to restrain an emotion even if it is legitimate and when to let it pour out.

Equipoise

While we might assume that meditation happens purely at the mental level, we can and do use meditation to cultivate the kind of equipoise in which we're not caught up in an emotion. Equipoise can be cultivated through a practice wherein a person discerns and recognizes a witnessing state, from which neutral observation can occur. I believe that is one of the essential steps in becoming a keen observer. Neutral observation does not imply apathy or indifference. Rather, it is a clear state of quiet observation in which it's possible to watch what arises. Guidance is given in the practice section for a basic meditation example.

Summary – Skillful Action

The message of the water element is learning how to be in flow. It is also a lesson of being what Charles calls *an agent of flow*. I like to think about this in some ways as being stuck in traffic. There are so many cars, all trying to get somewhere. You are sitting in a line of vehicles. A driver from an intersecting road would like to enter this line. You're presented with a choice: either you wave them in front of you or not. Either you can facilitate the need for another person to get to their destination, or you can choose not to help. The more we participate in the flow of life, supporting the cooperative effort to help everyone become aligned with and or stay on their path, the more fulfilling life becomes. Human beings are naturally inclined to nurture, to support, to help. Participation and cooperation are much more fundamental to human nature than many would believe. A river doesn't say to the fish that they can't be there.

Water element practice – Journal exercise

There are three cornerstones of practice that can help establish greater flexibility and flow with the water element. The first category falls under an age-old axiom of common sense, something Annie Besant identifies simply as "careful consideration before speech," one of the three methods she outlines for mastering emotions. The second category requires personal effort, which Annie Besant states is "the refusal to yield to impulse." In conjunction with a personal will, a decision is made inwardly to bring the emotions under one's control such that they become "useful servants instead of dangerous masters." The third category falls under the heading of "daily meditation" (Besant, A. p. 245). Meditation can take many forms. One essential component is the point or focus of concentration. The following exercise encompasses both a daily journal and a focal point in the form that we use. The focal point in the practice is the water element or emotional content. Mind and emotions are directly connected. Even though thought precedes feeling and feeling precedes emotion, a journaling exercise offers an opportunity to *empty out* the built-up emotions. In this way, built-up emotions are released rather than remaining stuck. Whenever you feel *stuck*, it is a signal that energy and life force are being blocked. The journaling exercise helps to develop and hold a witnessing state which is neutral. The writing medium performs the function of distance, creating space for participating in the exercise and simultaneously observing the words as they appear on the page. Journaling becomes a vehicle for disengaging from thought and emotion, opening the door of possibility, and seeing things in a new light.

To begin, find a place to sit that is relatively quiet and free of distraction. Place the notebook or paper in front of you or on your lap. Close your eyes. If you don't have a journal yet, start with a piece of paper. Use the next few moments to bring your attention to your breathing, lengthening your inhale and exhale for three rounds of breath. Now, open your eyes and take hold of the notebook or piece of paper. Think about the emotion that has arisen. Write it down, giving shape to the feeling such as *I feel sad* or *I feel angry*.

Next, write down any sensations you notice in your physical body that is associated with this emotion. If, for example, you feel sad, notice how the muscles of the face feel, whether the shoulders and chest feel open or sunken. Write down any other sensations you may have associated with the body. Next, ask inwardly as to why you feel this way. The process now opens the inquiry into the experience and what actions or experiences are related to the emotion. For example, it could be in reaction to something that someone said or did, or it could be that an event from a few days prior has not been fully processed. When emotions fill the mind, they usually turn into a story, often blocking the clarity needed for a higher perspective. The emotion is thus blocking the flow of life force and energy that would lead to clarity, insight, and understanding. Writing is, therefore, a medium that can help bring back the clarity needed. Keep writing until you have nothing left to write.

As the writing process is completed, notice the accompanying sensations. They may be a feeling of relief, calm, peacefulness, amongst others, as the journaling practice has ended for now. At this stage, sit quietly for a few minutes, integrating the sense of relief and lightness within yourself.

Later in the day or the next, you may want to review what you've written. It can be useful to examine whether or not your perspective has shifted, whether the emotion has cleared or is still present. Charged emotions indicate the need for more work to be done to clear them out. The journaling process can help dissolve charged or blocked emotions returning to a state of higher insight and understanding.

Going deeper

The first of the subtle elements to manifest is sound. It's no surprise then that music is such an important expression of human experience, connecting us to different parts of ourselves and connecting us to one other across space and time. One of my personal favorites is the sound of church bells. If I'm around when they're ringing, I'll usually stop whatever I'm doing to take in the melody briefly. Similarly, I love the chorus of voices singing in Gregorian chants and the slow rhythmic melodies of the Sitar and Esraj, musical instruments used in classical Indian music. Music has long played an important role in spiritual practice and rituals, such as chanting or singing hymns or prayers. Music and sound have a long history as a form of healing, such as sound therapy. According to Russill Paul, "the official term for the use of sound and music as a spiritual path is Nada Yoga, which literally translates as 'Sound Yoga'" (Paul, R. p. xiv).

Although we may think of music as the sound produced by the agency of an instrument(s), the human voice itself is an incredible instrument capable of producing a vast range of melodies. The human voice, whether producing sounds and melodies or repeating incantations and mantras, has a distinct role within the use of sound in healing and ritual. It has ancient roots which, as Russill Paul writes, "chanting is not a New Age fad; the use of sound as a means of yoga is grounded in traditions thousands of years old" (Paul, R. p. xiv).

Sound is all around us. In the Natural world, all birds have distinctive songs or melodies. Similarly, water produces a different sound when trickling gently along a brook versus gushing as a mountainous waterfall. As wood creaks under the heat of a fire, the embers crackle as the wood burns. Wind can sound like a high-speed train rushing through the trees or barely whispering as it glides over bare skin. Earth crunches underfoot in the dry decay of early winter or squishes and squeaks as boots sink into the mud. All sounds vibrate, at various frequencies, interacting within and around multiple energy fields. As we've examined in the book's structure, the human being is not just a physical body but a field of interpenetrating subtle bodies. And each subtle body vibrates at its own frequency. We can therefore think of music and or sound as a form for balancing the subtle energy bodies, healing where it's needed, and attuning the subtle bodies to the energies of the five elements.

One of my first introductions to using music connected with physical movement was as a young child learning ballet. I learned to cohesively integrate the various classical ballet steps as the pianist played for us. I'm still fond of the piano sonatas of Frédéric Chopin. Dance reveals that we can interpret thought, feeling, and emotion with music to tell a story. Like dance, combining music and bodywork therapy, it's possible to unfold the story wrapped in a person's body. Music can create a specific energetic tone for the space, music being a container for the healing session. Music can have a beneficial effect on many other movement disciplines, such as a yoga asana practice. Therefore, we can think about applying music and sound as a form for connecting us to the energies of the five elements in ourselves, in others, and around us. Through the agency of sound, we can fundamentally bring about a change in matter and consciousness, and to do that, we begin with intention. There are, therefore, two basic questions that are useful to keep in mind:

1. Direction/Focus – Which of the five elements needs to be amplified or pacified? For example, it could be to increase fire or decrease fire.

2. Setting – What is the environment in which the music is being applied? For example, a dental office versus a massage therapy or reiki office, or a yoga class versus a healing bodywork/energy-work session.

Working with direction and setting, you might start with the principle that an element represents. The next step involves selecting the sounds or music that most convey the energy of that element. Music choice should be tied to intention – considering what energy you want to facilitate shifting.

There's plenty of room to experiment where music and sound can be used as a practice that connects you to the five elements. As an example, you've spent the day heavily focused on a project involving hours in front of a computer. All this focus and concentration relies on the mind, which is the element of air. It can be restorative to sit down in a comfortable chair, listen to music, and reconnect and reground the physical body. It's not necessary to listen to a piece of recorded music either. You could sit beside a river listening to the different sounds the water makes as it glides over and around rocks, which provides a different experience of embodied groundedness. You could hear the sound a fire makes as wood crackles and creaks or pops loudly now and again, feeling increasingly more relaxed. It's important to keep in mind the relationship between the principle of the element and the qualities of the sound/music being used. Change is brought about when these are considered together rather than separately. The table below provides a beginning point for building a personal framework. The table shows connections between the principles and sound qualities to music with which you're most likely already familiar. Eventually, the framework can be expanded to include new music, developing a library composed of music and sounds. The examples offered in table 5.1 are from the library of music that I have used over the years. The range is diverse in genres – jazz, chanting, new age ambient, and classical. Samples of most if not all can be found online through the artists' websites directly or using other services such as Pandora, Spotify, or YouTube music.

Table 5.1 – Properties of sound.

Element	Principle	Sound qualities	Album/ Artist	Song
Earth	Grounding	Slow, steady, comforting	Garth Stevenson – *Flying*	"Dawn" and "Reflection"
			Jamie Lawrence – *At Ease*	"Meditation"
Water	Moving	Melodic, mellifluous, fluid	*From the Land of Ice and Snow – the songs of Led Zeppelin* (Various Artists)	Bron-Yr-Aur
Air	Elevating	Distant, mesmerizing, ambient, clarifying	Brian Eno – *Ambient 1: Music for Airports*	All songs on the album
Fire	Illuminating	Energizing, up-beat, vibrant	GoGo Penguin – *Man Made Object*	All songs on the album
Space	Emptiness	Silent, restful, blissful, tranquil	Craig Pruess and Ananda – *The Sacred Chants of Devi – 108 Sacred Names*	"Devi Prayer"

As you begin working with music for spiritual practice or healing, start with an intention or point of focus. For example, classical music has often been recommended to support students when they are studying for exams. Some of the music from this genre creates a state of consciousness that helps to elevate the students' minds to a state of clear focus and concentration, which is synonymous with a balanced air element. High energy exercise classes often utilize a lot of high tempo music, creating an atmosphere of excitement, motivation, and enthusiasm, all of which are qualities of the fire element. Spas and wellness centers usually have music piped throughout the center, creating an atmosphere that feels at once relaxing and grounding, inviting spa-goers to unwind stress and tension. This kind of music stimulates the connection to the groundedness of earth and the flow of water. As you play around and experiment with the music, notice the inner feelings and sensations that arise, making a point to acknowledge any changes you experience. In this way, it becomes possible to monitor inner growth and make adjustments toward creating inner balance, peace, and harmony.

Chapter 6

Air

Naturally, we may think of air primarily as the oxygen we breathe. However, examining the molecules and gases that form together to make air, we realize it has other properties besides its vital function of oxygenation for breathing and, thus, life. Air is the whole atmosphere of the planet, from the surface of the Earth outwards. Our atmosphere is composed of many layers. As we are investigating it, the element of air symbolizes the ability to look at things not just from above but really from a higher point of view. Relating this to each layer of our atmosphere, we could then say that each layer is like a different point along a spectrum, each of which would offer another point of view. The expression, "a thirty-thousand-foot view" suggests that by ascending to that height, a person can see a great distance down and wide, albeit not necessarily with a great level of detail. Just as you can ascend to a great height to get a better view, you can also zero in to get a closer, more detailed look at things.

In contrast, this means we can narrow our view to incredibly finite detail with something like a microscope. Air is a symbol for the expression of embodying lightness of being, which may be recognized as the ability to have a sense of humor and not take oneself too seriously. Lightness and humor are what give balance to perspective. Having a sense of humor does not mean that one laughs at the expense of someone else's pain or laughs off one's situation to avoid dealing with something difficult to acknowledge. It's natural to get stuck in a web of thoughts that dig the habit hole deeper rather than toward the light at the end of the tunnel. Sense of humor provides a new way to see a situation, oneself, or someone else, creating an opportunity to be lifted or to lift others.

Life is an endless series of possibilities, of seeing life as one experiment after the next. You try something, it doesn't work, so you try something else. The stickiness comes in when any endeavor that you take on is thought of as the only possibility, the only way, that if it fails or doesn't work, it means the end of all other options. These are all erroneous views. We can increase mental flexibility and keep life force flowing by cultivating a mindset that recognizes the unlimited possibilities available and that as one door appears to close, another opens. The opposite is a quagmire of mental stagnation like a hot day with air so thin you can hardly think about moving in one direction or another.

As we stated earlier, the air element represents perspective. As the source of the beliefs and values that each person holds, the mental body shapes the worldviews through which each individual sees the world – their own and others. The manifested reality is shaped and formed through these various viewpoints, rooted in core beliefs and values. We don't just experiment with projects but also with belief systems to see what fits with our values and what doesn't. In the same way that air can become stale in an unventilated room, beliefs themselves can become stagnant and rigid. A room needs to be ventilated for air to move, to be refreshed and renewed. Air element, therefore, teaches us that our beliefs are not some rigid concrete structures. Rather, beliefs and viewpoints are malleable. As we learn to harness the power of the mind, we increase our ability to adapt our thinking, which has a positive benefit not just for an individual but also globally. A mind that is stable and capable of holding different points of view without judgment is also capable, therefore, of seeing others from their point of view. A mind of equipoise is an essential component of cultivating compassion, which is the ability to see someone else in their unique situation with as little of your own bias as possible and be open-hearted and kind to their suffering. All the world benefits when each of us is willing and able to see one another from a higher perspective.

The mind is associated with the air element because a function of the mind is the ability to analyze, categorize, direct focus, direct attention, and process sensory data as input and output.

The difficulty in directing this executive function is where human beings are endowed with a personality and ego. In the most basic terms, the ego likes to be in control, and the personality has many things it likes and many things it doesn't like. These two human attributes can shift a person's view from a mode of neutral observation to a mode of judgment, whether positive or negative. The personality has polarized the point of view. As we'll see a little later in the book, neutral observation, and non-judgmental insight comes from the illumination of a higher level of being, namely from the soul.

In general, though, we could say that erroneous views are like clouds: a clear blue sky is obscured on a cloudy day, and erroneous views obscure clear thinking. In essence, expressions such as *clouded thinking* or *cloudy judgment* describe an air element that is not in balance, the opposite of mental equipoise. As Obi-Wan Kenobi says to his student in *Star Wars Episode VI – Return of the Jedi* (1983), "Luke, you're going to find that many of the truths we cling to depend greatly on our own point of view."

Contemplation

We all need time and space to gather our thoughts, time to reflect, and be still. Think about the value of taking time out after situations like these:

1. An important conversation covering a lot of detailed information
2. A challenging discussion trying to resolve a conflict
3. A long lecture in which new and unfamiliar details were covered

4. A class that now challenges you to expand on prior knowledge and which requires assimilation of old with new

Three ways to support the need for contemplation involves:

1. Integration
2. Open-mindedness
3. Quiet time

In essence, the volume of information or data needs to go through several steps before it can be integrated and for decisions or choices to be made. These steps involve absorption or taking in, processing, sorting (categorizing and organizing), and assessment. A formalized process such as journaling and writing until there is a natural impulse to stop, a signal that a break is needed, or there's nothing further to write can support the integration process. This act of writing can remove the clouds floating around in the head. It can be easier to review and examine thoughts once written on paper.

Cultivating an open mind also means needing to consider differing or complementary points of view. In this sense, contemplation involves actively choosing an unfamiliar subject to expand your thinking. For instance, comparative studies of different world religions would fall under this heading.

We also need time and space to quiet the mind, which could be facilitated by sitting outside surrounded by Nature, without engaging in thoughts and listening inwardly. Meditation is another method, using techniques that help disengage thoughts from arising, moving into a state of clear tranquility and calm abiding.

Connection

We all need to spend time with people with whom we have shared values and beliefs. The people we spend time with regularly and with whom close connections are shared are more enjoyable and supportive when we each are on the same or similar wavelength. Not only are conversations more engaging and fulfilling, but shared activities also provide an opportunity to express this connection. For instance, you and a friend may both love visiting museums with a special emphasis on painters from the early twentieth century. Or you may participate in volunteer work together that focuses on raising awareness of climate change.

Raising consciousness

Mentally engaging and stimulating experiences fall under this heading. These experiences are uplifting, expand thinking and understanding, and may even lead to pursuing new experiences, increasing flexibility of consciousness. Elevating consciousness also involves reading text or scripture that brings one closer to the light of illuminated thinking and the soul's light and illumination. Sources could include reading beautiful poetry, sacred scripture, or especially poignant verses from a play. The source material is not only uplifting; it opens the heart and softens a little more of the illusory boundaries of separation.

Summary – Skill in Action

A view is just a view. A belief is just a belief. A point of view is just a point of view. A flexible mind realizes that life is always changing – the more flexible the mind, the greater the experience of inner freedom. Anytime we cling to a view or belief as if it were an irreplaceable treasure, stuckness and stagnation arise, even pain and suffering. The skill of a balanced air element is adjusting course like the winds that carry change and realizing that forms are always dissolving and emerging.

Breath practice

An essential component of quieting the mind is the breath. Regulating the breath has the effect of calming and slowing down the mind. In turn, breath and mind become synchronized, which opens the door to the realms of inner peace and inner joy. We don't ever think about breathing, not consciously anyway. It's an involuntary body function that we're able to bring under voluntary control. In virtually all beginner meditation exercises, meditators are instructed to start with the breath. And, all longtime meditators, including the ones that I know, use the breath to begin a meditation session. Therefore, breath practice is not just for beginners but provides constant support that steadies a long-term commitment to regular and ongoing meditation practice.

Just as breath is an essential component of meditation, so is posture essential for easy breathing. The way the body is positioned and then held for the duration of the meditation session influences one's ability to remain focused on the task at hand. Maintaining the single-pointed focus is more easily accomplished if the mind is not also distracted by the niggles and wiggles of the body. Patanjali's Yoga Sūtras place *āsana* (which can mean posture or seat) as the third rung in an eight-stepped ladder, placing this before *pranayama* (breath exercise) and the four successive stages of meditation. Asana is especially useful for modern bodies – a modern lifestyle that generally tends toward being more sedentary and repetitive in the tasks such as sitting at a desk for eight hours. Movement practices such as Hatha Yoga that emphasize both the strength and flexibility of the body provide a good foundation for the static and steady posture that is necessary for meditation. In the exercise described below, posture is taken to mean a relatively stationary position that the body inhabits for the duration of the practice. There are three options in which this can be done: sitting, standing, or lying down. For this practice, we outline what is needed for sitting, whether on the floor or in a chair.

We begin by positioning the body such that the hips feel open and the legs through the knees are relaxed and at ease.

The pelvis should be somewhat neutral, neither tilted such that the lower back is excessively arched nor tucked such that the lower back is overly flat. The back should be upright with a feeling of length that reaches upward, providing the necessary space for the entire chest to open and expand. (As a contrast, you could slouch or slump for a moment to feel the difference.) It can be useful to imagine the spine for a moment as something like a string of pearls. Each vertebra is like a pearl with inherent strength and vitality. There is a little space between each one so that they stack gracefully one above the other. The thread holding them together is like silk – incredibly strong and simultaneously flexible. Keeping the back upright should feel strong, flexible, and relaxed rather than rigid and heavy. The arms hang loosely, which is easier by placing the hands on the legs either separately or by resting one hand in the other. The head is held upright, gazing forward, with a very gentle and slight nod downward. Lightly bring the lips together, unclenching the jaw as you do so. The face is open, soft, relaxed. As the posture becomes settled, imagine the tension and the activities of the day draining out of the body. Now we may continue with the rest of the practice.

Closing your eyes, turn your attention and mental focus inward. Realize that you are breathing, feeling the expansion and contraction of the diaphragm, the rising and falling of the chest and abdomen. Consciously begin to lengthen the breath. Slowly deepen the inhale and deepen the exhale. Repeat this process of taking long slow breaths, without strain or force. Keep the flow of the breath steady and easeful. You may realize how absorbed your focus and concentration have been for the last few minutes. Continue to deepen your concentration with each breath. Start equalizing the breath, lengthening the inhale and exhale. It could be two to three seconds for each inhale and exhale, or longer such as three to five seconds. Duration will depend on your breath capacity and should not be forced or strained in any way. Continue at your own pace, maintaining the same steady concentration and focus on the breath. After three minutes have elapsed, bring your breath back to its regular rhythm. Notice the changes in your awareness, your perception of the room you're in, the sensations of your body, your mind's ability to remain relatively steady and focused, and how you feel. Take a few more moments to gather this information. Gradually, open your eyes, returning to the regular waking consciousness focus. Move around and stretch the body a bit. You may want to consider keeping a journal to record your experiences as you develop this foundational practice. It's a good idea to repeat this practice daily for at least one month, an average rule of thumb when attempting to change a habit or develop a new one.

Practice – Seeing the mind as a calm, clear lake

Perspective is hard to come by when the mind is turbulent. Meditation practices such as this are an important step in developing the capacity to remain clear and present in especially challenging moments. The practice cultivates a certain kind of resilience to external and internal stressors that would take us off our center and cloud the mind. The metaphor in this practice uses the image of a calm, clear lake to symbolize what the mind is like in its natural state. In this way, and with the associated imagery, we may be better able to conceptualize and orient ourselves to this state of consciousness not just once but repeatedly.

To begin the practice, settle into a comfortable seated position. Align your body in a meditation posture, equal weight through the pelvis, upright back, open chest, softness in the face, head bowed slowly downward. Close the eyes, drawing attention and focus inward. Settle the mind by focusing on the breath; long and steady inhales and exhales. With the breath slowing down, invite the body to follow along. With each exhale, imagine the activities of the day draining out as if you had just washed the body in a shower. With each inhale, imagine the body growing lighter and more spacious from the inside. After a minute or so, turn your attention to the center of your forehead. Imagine a point extending as a straight line from the center of your forehead to a spot about five feet in front of you. That spot marks a location in the middle of a mental landscape — finding a clearing through surrounding trees at the edge of a lake. As you walk up to the water's edge, notice how still and calm the surface of the water is. The water is so calm that it perfectly reflects the light of the sun and a few passing clouds from above. Hold your attention here on the lake for a while longer. Know that you can return to this place at any time. Instead of turning your back on the water as you would if you were hiking away, draw yourself back along the line that extends from the center point of your forehead. Watch as the lake gradually becomes smaller until it's no longer visible, the image fading gently. Return the focus of your attention to your breath so that it may re-anchor you in the body. After drawing the meditation to a close, open the eyes after a few moments, eventually stretching the body with simple movements.

As stated in the previous exercise above, practice daily for at least one month, an average rule of thumb when attempting to change a habit or develop a new one.

Journal practice

This practice involves sitting down to write with the express intention to empty your mind of the thoughts keeping you in a state of stagnation rather than flow. Writing begins with the first thing that comes to mind, without judging what you have written or may be about to write. As each thought comes to mind, you write it down. After a few minutes, you may find that the words are flowing onto the pages. When there is nothing further to write, you stop. Before you read what you have written, pause to close your eyes and notice how you feel. How has your experience of your energy changed? How has your experience of your body changed? How has the perception of your surroundings changed? Emptying the mind is like emptying a bucket of sand. A bucket of sand is heavy. When the bucket is empty, it is light, having barely any weight compared to when it was filled with sand moments before. The more you familiarize yourself with the feeling of lightness and emptiness, the easier it becomes to return to this state, until eventually, this becomes the default.

Going deeper

A selection of various sutras, aphorisms, passages, and quotes are offered here for your reflection and meditation. Select only one at a time and not necessarily in the sequence in which they are presented here. When reading a passage, notice the energy behind the words. The invitation here is to *feel into* what you are reading, rather than simply analyzing the words for what they mean. The words contain an energy and the energy of the individual who wrote or translated them. As you feel into the words, close your eyes and let the feeling guide your state of focus. Think of the selected passage or phrase as containing a particular state of consciousness. As you meditate on the words and the feeling behind them, you open yourself up to the state of consciousness itself. All that anyone can ever really do is point to a path and try to shed some light. As you meditate, you are not trying to replicate any particular achievement or replicable experience. You will experience the state of consciousness in your unique way.

"The practice of meditation frees one from all affliction. This is the path of yoga. Follow it with determination and sustained enthusiasm. Renouncing wholeheartedly all selfish desires and expectations, use your will to control the senses. Little by little, through patience and repeated effort, the mind will become stilled in the Self" (Easwaran, E. p. 145).

"Cultivate vigor, patience, will, purity; avoid malice and pride. Then, Arjuna, you will achieve your divine destiny" (Easwaran, E. p. 238).

"When the five senses of perception along with the mind are at rest, and even the intellect has ceased functioning, That, sages say, is the Supreme state" (Saraswati, 2004. p.139).

Chapter 7

Mind

Your thoughts become your words. From your words, you develop your actions. From your actions you create your reality.

The first time I came across this concept was probably some time in my early twenties. Like the sound of church bells that ring loudly and clearly, it completely captured my attention. It felt as though the power of the words had pierced a veil, a feeling of familiarity that I couldn't quite place yet rang as true and as clear, just like the church bells. Although I felt a veil being pierced, the hole itself was small, more like a tiny pinprick versus a gaping crater. But, that first hole was just big enough to allow in a ray of light, the light that reflects a deep knowing and the recognition of something completely timeless. I didn't yet have a grasp of the enormity of what it truly meant, yet this tiny seed of powerful wisdom stayed with me. As the years passed, variations of this original Upanishad would appear, either quoted or reframed in some way. One such reframing had a powerful impact on me. It happened when I began reading a book called *The Nature of Personal Reality*. Seth, a non-physical teacher, channeled by Jane Roberts, made a simple statement: **You make your own reality** (Roberts, J. p. 20). It was typed in bold, as it is here. The words seemed to reach off the pages and grab me, shaking me awake. The tiny hole from years earlier was now blown wide open. I realized two things. First, I could create my own reality by harnessing the power of my mind. Second, I alone was responsible for creating that reality. Although I had this insight, there was still a lot more information I needed to understand how this actually worked. As I turned back to the philosophy of yoga and the Upanishads, over time, I found an elegant framework that could explain some of the deeper inner workings of how thought and mind function. Guidance from my spiritual mentor and the written teachings of others proved to be indispensable, especially where some of the philosophies were more obscure or did not explicitly provide a step-by-step set of instructions for how to practice.

Knowing and understanding the nature of the mind is, well, not all that easy. The mind can be quite elusive, like wisps of smoke that you try to hold with your hands. Similarly, it can be just as ephemeral to describe the mind, hence the many books that exist trying to do just that. This chapter attempts to describe the mind and its fundamental nature while providing some exercises and practices for your exploration. However, I would add a caution that working with the mind should not be a solitary endeavor. It is essential to have a mentor, advisor, trusted friend, or community. One element of studying the mind is realizing that every individual has at least one if not more blindspots. It is something in your own psyche you cannot see or may not want to see. People want to meditate; possibly have experiences of an enlightenment. However, the question is this, "Are you willing to do the inner work needed to be prepared for higher states of consciousness?" Therefore, this chapter could be considered a simple introduction to the nature of the mind, one which may provide some basic foundational structure that can be built upon.

Liberation

Before we examine the nature of the mind, it is important to consider the motivation for this undertaking as something other than an intellectual pursuit.

Liberation is understood as two things. First, it is the innate power to free oneself from illusion. Illusion is twofold:

1. The misidentification of the real Self as the false self.
2. The obscurations caused by the part of the mind that creates the veil of illusion and thus suffering.

Second, liberation is understood as freeing oneself from the repetitive cycle of cause and effect – karma.

"The source of liberation, self-liberation, and inner freedom, is within one's own ability and power. It is an 'intrapsychic event, not a locality'" (Feuerstein, G. p. 229). With the right understanding and set of appropriate tools, it is possible to live from the power of conscious thought and action, a "shift in consciousness whereby one transcends all duality" (Feuerstein, G. p. 230). Otherwise, an untamed mind is like a train without a conductor – without direction and control, the train risks going too fast and even off the tracks.

Locus of Mind

The evolution of an individual, as we normally think of, begins from the time the transcendent Self individuates from the Source right up to the moment it becomes physically embodied. In between all these unfolding stages is what could be thought of as the halfway point. At this halfway point, the *ātman* comes into being. [A small "a" in *ātman* denotes the false self, whereas a capital "A" would denote the true Self.] Coming into being is not so much one single stage but a series and, in a sense, begins when the mind is formed. Therefore, we can think of this as the formless aspect of the transcendent Self meeting the part of itself that takes form, which is atman, at the halfway point, which is the mind. Although it can seem as though the mind is like a black box – stuff goes in, and stuff comes out, but what happens inside the black box is a bit of a mystery; it's actually more like a totally clear and unblemished crystal. The crystal simply reflects whatever is projected onto it. The mind is, therefore, like a clearinghouse that receives, processes, and transmits information from the *atman* down into physical reality and back up again. The transmission of this passing information back and forth is nothing other than the process of learning and growth. However, the process itself can be very sticky and quite murky if the mind is not clear and if a good supervisor is not there to watch over things. Within the clearinghouse, there are logistics centers, and these are the components of the mind we examine next.

Components of Mind

In general, the typical idea of the mind has been to see it as a function of the brain; chemical processes, memory. Indian philosophy, however, conceives of the mind as a function beyond the physical body but which is necessary for the transcendent Self to navigate within physical reality. There are three main operators of the logistics center, continuing with our analogy from above:

1. Buddhi – intelligence, knowledge, and wisdom of the soul
2. Ahamkāra – the false self as ego/personality
3. Manas – subjective reality experienced as feelings, emotions, beliefs

These three principles together comprise the mental operations, the framework of which is the same in each individual.

Buddhi

Buddhi is a psycho-spiritual assembly of higher capacities: wisdom, intuition, discernment, insight and perspicuity. Once the mind is illuminated from *buddhi*, it is experienced simultaneously as clear and luminous. In a way, *buddhi* lights up what is already there – the nature of the mind in its restful and pure state. More than even a clear crystal, the mind itself is like a rare unblemished diamond. A well-known property of a diamond is its ability to cut through just about anything; so powerful is its inherent strength. Ultimately, *buddhi* illuminates the diamond-like nature of the mind, which cuts through all illusions. Thus, it can be thought of as the "higher mind." Although *buddhi* is bright like the sun, it can be obscured in similar terms to the phenomenon of a solar eclipse. Whereas a solar eclipse may last only a few minutes, mental obscurations may block the radiance of the mind for much longer.

In practical terms, experiencing the mind as clear and luminous usually occurs due to training the other aspects of the mind. One example is meditation which teaches how to cultivate attention in single-pointed concentration. Beginning meditators typically start a practice of mindfulness of the breath. Most people quickly realize how difficult it is to maintain an uninterrupted focus on the breath. The mind is quickly and easily distracted, more like a wild horse than one tamed by its rider. Gradually, mind training exercises become progressively more challenging.

Another example is meditation to train the senses. In this type of concentration practice, a meditator learns to disengage from the senses that are trying to distract attention. Instead of turning awareness to listen attentively to birds singing outside, the focus would be directed to disengage from the sound. The sound falls away, more like a backdrop to the task at hand. As the mind becomes more stable, less like an untamed wild horse, it's possible to draw in this light of higher wisdom, cutting through one illusion after another such that glimpses of the diamond-like quality of the mind become more and more visible.

Ahamkara – Ego-Personality

Ahamkara is essentially the fabricated self. It's fabricated because it believes itself to be the real self, the head honcho, the commander-in-chief. As the ego-personality, it's forgotten what its function is. It has confused itself, but rather than recognizing the confusion; it reinforces its belief that *it* is in charge. Day after day, it reinforces this belief. The ego-personality caught in its own illusion, does not realize itself to be a part of the mind. In a sense, this powerful self-generated illusion eclipses the radiance of the mind, the light, and wisdom shining through from the unlimited Self. Suffering then, seen from this perspective, is the result of forgetting the real Self.

The ego-personality is meant to function as a wise general in the captain's army. Instead of taking direction, however, from the captain, it is constantly trying to wage a mutiny to wrestle control. The wise general is afraid that the captain will try to send it to the gallows to meet its final demise. However, it does not realize that the captain has no such intention. The captain needs the general. If it were to let go of control, its greatest fear would be realized – annihilation. And this presents a common misunderstanding in which it's believed that you need to cut off the head of the ego to be free from it and, therefore, to realize the true Self. Not only is this not true, but not possible. You cannot get rid of the ego-personality. Rather, you, as captain, need to transcend your attachment to the ego-personality, the wise general in your command. It's the attachment that causes part of the confusion and reinforces the ego-personality's belief that it's the real self. The ego-personality serves an important function. Ego is the part of us that needs motivation and drive in order to be propelled forward in the process of unfolding a lifetime.

The personality is that part of each of us that creates the unique variety of identities that make a rainbow constellation of individuals all on a collective journey. Attachment to the ego-personality is both the identity of who we believe ourselves to be and all the self-imposed limitations that obscure living from the radiant beauty of the true Self. Those limitations are a vast collection, including the lifetime of social and family conditioning, limiting beliefs, beliefs, and values that are inconsistent with each other, unresolved past experiences, and more. One mechanism that perpetuates the notion of a limited self is that when it's stuck in its own illusion, the ego-personality is ruled by desire for that which increases pleasure and that which decreases pain. A simpler way to conceive of this is simply as likes and dislikes. Likes and dislikes tend to be entrenched thoughts and behaviors, not always obvious in their appearance. They can be quite dogmatic, too, further reinforcing the pattern. Likes and dislikes are two of five major mechanisms that drive illusions, which we examine in the next section.

Mind/Manas

Indian philosophy and the language of Sanskrit, has a nuanced and subtle conceptual framework of the mind. For instance, distinctions are made with the faculty that synthesizes information (*manas*) versus the faculty that uses discernment and wisdom (*buddhi*). There is a distinction made between thoughts and thinking versus awareness and consciousness. In this section, manas is that aspect of the mind that synthesizes information, processing and organizing into categories. As we experience the world, whether the world is outside of ourselves or our interior inner world, the experiences are processed by way of the five senses. One category is the knowledge senses (*pancha jñānendriya*):

1. Auditory – sound/hearing
2. Vision – sight
3. Tactile – touch
4. Gustation – taste
5. Olfaction – smell

The other category is the action senses (*pancha karmmendriya*):

1. Speech, communication, and expression
2. Movement and locomotion

3. Grasping and maneuverability
4. Emission and procreation
5. Digestion and elimination

As incoming information is recorded, it is converted into familiar concepts and images. When the senses make contact with external phenomena, that contact is recorded as activities that increase pleasure and decrease pain. Attaching a label to the data is, you could say, a last step. The labels are mental "feelings"; a tree might be recorded simply as "tree." But, if you are someone with seasonal allergies, the tree might be labeled as "unpleasant" or "disliked" even if it's not the source of the allergic reaction.

As we examine this last stage of labeling more deeply, we find that "pleasure" and "pain" can be sub-divided into more specialized categories. This is useful in that it enables us to more easily clarify where the mind is stuck and caught in its own web. Categories are operational modes – the way the lower mind captures, sorts, analyzes, processes, and records data from activities. These modes are the modes of obscuration, outlined below beginning, with the *kleshas*. As with medicine, we need to understand the root cause of something in order for the application of an antidote to be truly effective. This is a gradual process – there is no quick fix. Expecting immediate results only serves to entrench the illusions further.

The senses are generally active all the time; data is constantly being recorded, some of which we are typically not aware of in the moment. That would be too much information to process in any one given moment. Lower mind is, therefore, always quite busy. When the lower mind is described as being *like a monkey*, this refers to the constant activity of processing data without the ability or awareness to disengage. In other words, when left untrained, the senses constantly swing like a monkey from one experience to another. This constant activity can be quite tiring.

And much like the chatter of a group of monkeys, so too is a busy mind noisy. This mental noise is composed of thoughts, feelings, and emotions which arise based on how the senses have recorded various activities. This recording process is generally termed mental obscurations. What has been obscured is reality, and all obscurations become some form of obstacle and limitation. Eventually, all limitations need to be burned up in the fire of higher wisdom, where they may become the spiritual fuel for furthering the continued evolution of learning and growth. Burning away the limitations is, ultimately, self-liberation.

Five obscurations and fabrications of mental perception called kleshas are outlined in Patanjali's Yoga Sūtras. Similar to the concept of Buddhism's *five poisons*, kleshas are hindrances that are meant to be overcome to simultaneously free oneself from the seeds that produce karma and see the light of the true Self. The kleshas are:

1. Avidyā – Ignorance; lack of spiritual knowledge
2. Asmitā – Ego/Personality; the generation of the sense of the false "I"
3. Rāga – Attachment to that which causes pleasure; desire
4. Dveṣaḥ – Aversion to that which causes pain; fear, dislike
5. Abhiniveśāḥ – Fear of death; clinging in various forms including to life

In practice, an individual gradually works moment-to-moment to dissolve the obscurations, lessening the degree to which there is the experience of displeasure/pain/suffering and increasing the thoughts and actions which increase satisfaction, fulfillment, and joy.

As obscurations are gradually worn away, it becomes like cleaning dust off a mirror. As the dust is wiped away, the mirror does not dissolve but instead shines. Without any impurities to cover it, the mirror is able to reflect what is truly there, which is the mind reflecting itself in its pure state. As mental obscurations are dissolved, the pristine natural state of the mind becomes visible. This natural state is one of tranquil and quiescent luminosity. It's possible to see the mind this way as consciousness – the mind has the special capability to turn awareness in the direction of becoming aware of itself. It also means it has the ability to experience its own luminosity and to witness itself, as in the relationship of subject and object. An analogy I often use to describe this state is the experience of observing a lake on a calm day. The water is brilliantly crystal clear, and with the absence of wind or any other movement, the water remains near-perfectly motionless. The motionless state of the water grants it the appearance of being both glass-like and mirror-like. Light from the sun above penetrates through all the layers of the water unimpeded until it reaches the sand at the bottom. With the surface of the water motionless, it reflects the sun back to itself – the sun able to see itself in the reflection of the water. Obscurations of the mind block the light of higher wisdom and inner illumination. Therefore, examining each category is a step toward removing whatever it is that blocks that light for oneself.

Ignorance/Avidya

By definition, ignorance is a lack of knowledge, unconsciousness, or a lack of awareness. Lack of knowledge is taken to mean the true Self. Secondly, and just as importantly, it is the misperception of life as permanent and unchanging. Human beings are conditioned by their experiences. More broadly, this can be thought of under the heading of "family and social conditioning." In general, the misperception of conditioned experiences is believing them to define who someone is, including oneself. Conditioned experience is shaped via the set of beliefs that a person chooses, consciously or unconsciously, which shapes their worldview. Misperception then, seen from this perspective, is not knowing that beliefs do change and can change. Realizing the true Self is, in part, realizing that a person is not inherently their beliefs.

The antidote to avidya is to be curious and to inquire. Curiosity engages the learning process with an open mind. It's an invitation to ask questions and to follow the voice that wonders and imagines. It is also the courage to admit to what you don't yet know while simultaneously summoning the motivation and willingness to take steps to learn. Human beings eventually learned that the Earth was not flat but round because someone dared to challenge that long-held belief.

Sense of "I"/Asmita

The fabricated self, the ego/personality, believes itself to be the real self. It becomes caught up in its own web, reifying the sense of "I" and believing it to be the real self. The I-maker, *ahamkara*, as it sometimes called (the ego principle), does not realize that it is the false self. As it tries to maintain control, it has the ability to effectively "wall-out" the voice of the real Self, the true recognition of the real Self. On the other hand, the "pure-I" is the part of consciousness that split off from and separated itself from the Source. In general, this pure-I is "forgotten" and needs to be re-remembered and re-recognized. This re-cognition is possible because the inherent memory of the "pure-I" is maintained within the separated individual Self that is created. Let's imagine for a moment that we've parked our car in a really large parking lot or garage. We return some hours later, having no memory whatsoever of where the car is now parked. We hope that this loss of memory of where the car is parked is just temporary. We mentally retrace our steps and try to think of landmarks and, less helpfully, the color or models of other cars. If we happen to recall the memory, we may jump, even if only in our own head, in joyful relief. Sometimes, we wander row by row, level by level, until the car is located at last. In this hypothetical example, the car represents the object-side of our innate Self, one which is used for navigating the ups and downs of learning and growth. Remembering where the car is located described one moment in a series of moments in which the essence of the true Self is recalled, recollected, and re-remembered. The car was not lost; it was simply unavailable to our primary waking consciousness.

Attachment (rāga) and aversion (dvesha)

Attachment and aversion are simply versions of desire and fear, likes and dislikes, pleasure and pain. As the five senses record sense impressions and sense data, they go through the filter of the ego-personality (ahamkara), which has a desire to create experiences that increase pleasure and decrease pain. In general, this can be thought of as sense data being recorded as either something that is liked or something that is disliked. Unlike preferences which are more flexible and less fixed and have the flexibility and willingness to adapt and change, likes and dislikes are entrenched habits of processing and categorizing experiences. They can be so habitual that, more often than not, we don't realize the extent to which our experiences are labeled and sorted in this way. The more rigid likes and dislikes become, the more likely they are to block the natural flow of vitality and life force, much like plaque builds up in arteries which block the vital flow of blood to the heart. This way of thinking generally polarizes thoughts, narrowing the point of view. In some cases, a perspective can become so narrow as to reach its extreme. True and lasting satisfaction is never fully realized or experienced when the habit of this entrenched mode of recording experiences and trying to create reality continues operating. Likes and dislikes feed each other so that it becomes a never-ending loop. You run toward what you desire and hold on as tightly as you can when you have it because you fear losing it. What you fear will rarely happen, but then you draw the fear to yourself through obsessive worrying, and then you run as fast as you can. In this continual loop, change and growth can often stagnate.

Fundamentally, all of created reality is an expression of the Universal impulse to create, to will into being some creative expression of a kind of manifested reality. At the highest level, it is the impulse of the Source, of their will and desire, to manifest a Universe. This will and desire are mirrored in the impulse to create a reality that expresses one's own individuality in an individual. The fundamental misunderstanding is trying to create reality through a misapplication of personal will. This personal will is filled with lots of expectations and demands, attachment and craving, fear and worry. In any area where it is perceived that personal will is being blocked, an experience will be labeled/recorded as "not liking" or "dislike." Similarly, trying to exert personal will to get what is perceived to increase happiness, an experience will be labeled/recorded as "like" or "want more of." Neither of these states produces lasting satisfaction, and more often than not, create suffering for oneself and others.

The antidote to *likes* and *dislikes* is the ability to move fluidly, from one experience to the next, moment to moment. In practice, we are cultivating the skill to free ourselves from the control of the five senses. When the senses no longer control how we approach or inhabit an experience, there's much more freedom to open to the flow of the experience as it unfolds in the moment. And often, to our amazement, a magical sense of joy and satisfaction arises.

When I first met my husband, he had offered to prepare dinner for us, with one of the main ingredients being green beans. I had long ago placed green beans into the *dislike* category. As a result, I never actively shopped for them nor looked for recipes for how to cook them. I actively stayed away from them. Despite my strong dislike for green beans, I was willing to try them in this circumstance. Besides, he'd already demonstrated on prior occasions that he was a good cook! Much to my surprise, I found the dish to be highly enjoyable. I also realized that green beans could be really delicious when freshly picked and prepared well. No soggy green beans here! It's now become something I enjoy with much satisfaction.

Whether it's food or another kind of experience, the key is being open to the opportunity to try something new and, in the process, learn and grow. Rather than being constrained and limited by strongly held *likes* and *dislikes*, we return to a state of flexibility when approaching life with curiosity and a willingness to explore.

Fear of death or clinging to life/Abhinivesah

Under this heading, there are three categories:

1. Clinging to the false self – spiritual death, the ego needs to be integrated.
2. Clinging to the false body – physical death in which the body dies and consciousness continues, reincarnates.
3. Clinging to experience – all experiences undergo cycles of birth/emergence, manifestation/maintenance, and dissolution/death.

The fabricated self clings to experiences in the first category because it believes itself to be the real Self. Its greatest fear is the fear of death, which is rooted in the notion that life is completely extinguished (annihilation) once consciousness leaves the body. Clinging tightly to this false self in the second category is an attempt to hold on as tightly as possible to the body and anything material. The belief is that the material is real and lasting, a deeply held illusion and misperception that all life is impermanent. If you live in the moment, present to all that is, and in dialogue with your true Self, the more life force you allow to flow through you to all levels of being. It is then possible to experience life as magical, the nirvana of being in the here and now. The fear of allowing experiences in the third category to dissolve and change form is clinging to them even when they have already long passed. All things in the universe are in a state of unfolding and dissolving, taking form, becoming an experience, and then eventually dissolving and or changing form. We can see these cycles of manifestation in everyday life such as:

- the ending of a relationship
- the closing of a business
- the sale of a house
- the loss of a job or starting a new one
- the changing of careers
- the change of the seasons
- a plant losing an old leaf as a new one emerges

The process of dissolving allows something new to emerge, which reflects the natural order of the Universe, constantly in a state of expansion and contraction, unfolding and returning. Clinging to any experience, whether it be the desire for something wanted or unwanted, leads to the experience of suffering. Death is not an ending but a doorway into new possibilities. There are three antidotes to clinging that free up the mind from fear, taking another step closer toward joy. These are:

1. **Impermanence**. All things and all phenomena are impermanent. States of mind change, emotions rise and fall away, the body changes every second, producing new cells as old cells die and are replaced. The seasons of nature change.
2. **Self-study**. Learning all there is to know about oneself is a lifetime study. We work with all parts of ourselves in

the process, including those we might not like to see. As we engage in self-discovery, we peel back the layers that obscure the true Self.

3. **Curiosity**. Turning fear into curiosity fuels the learning process. One place to start is with an "if" statement. For example, "what if I tried this?" Or, "what is needed of me in this moment?" Questions like these open a dialogue between the ego and the soul, drawing in more life force and openness to more possibilities.

Confusion

Although the mind state of confusion is not listed within Patanjali's model of the five *kleshas*, it is something most people experience at one time or another. And it can be tricky to figure out how to extract yourself from it. Confusion, from this perspective, is thus a sixth klesha or obstacle. The challenge with confusion is how the mind becomes stuck. Adding to the difficulty is that the harder you try not to be confused, the more it's reinforced! Instead of mental freedom, there's a state of limbo – there is no movement in any direction. Energy and life force become stagnant, even blocked. Keep in mind that confusion is a mind state rather than an emotion. Emotions may arise eventually, particularly the longer the confusion lasts, such as frustration or anger.

The best way out of confusion is to reach for a higher perspective, which is the soul's insight. Charles has offered this definition of confusion as "not accepting the pictures of reality that are being shown or reflected." What is meant by this statement is that the mind holds one picture, and reality holds another. The mind refuses to accept a picture that differs from the one it's currently holding. Confusion arises when these two images cannot be reconciled. If we take the definition offered above and turn it into a practice, we have a mechanism for drawing in the soul's insight and extracting ourselves from our confusion.

The first step is to acknowledge that you are feeling confused. The next step is to remind yourself of what creates the confusion. Drawing on Charles's definition, inwardly repeat, as if calling upon a mantra: "confusion is not accepting the pictures of reality that are being shown to me." In the third step, draw a line down the center using a piece of paper or journal. On one side, write down your thoughts and feelings. You can, of course, also draw a picture if you like. On the other side, write down what reality is showing you – then compare the two. A slight variation on this practice is turning the statement into a question: "what picture of reality am I not accepting?"

As you work through the question, making comparisons if you have opted to write down your experience, it is useful to examine some of the roots of the confusion. The issue of not accepting a picture of reality that is different is essentially rooted in attachment and expectation – to something or someone. Although it is only mentioned in the scripture three times, the Bhagavad Gita offers brief but sage counsel for just this situation. The first begins with controlling the senses (Sūtra 2.63), the primary doorway in which external objects are contacted. Craving for and desire for material things only brings temporary happiness. When happiness does not last, the mind is confused – the material thing was meant to bring lasting happiness, but it didn't. Sense control is realizing the temporary and changing nature of all things. Second, similar to what has been stated earlier involves drawing upon the insight and knowledge from the higher Self or soul (Sūtra 4.35). When our daily waking or ordinary focused consciousness is infused with the light of the soul, or *buddhi*, the perspective of reality is illuminated from a higher point of view. This state of consciousness is reached not from wishing or hoping but through sincere and dedicated effort to remove all the obscurations that conceal the true Self. Practices that develop this in meditation have at their foundation re-remembering the distinction between the true Self and the false self; the witness and the participant; the observer and the observed (Sūtra 13.6).

The way out of confusion begins with curiosity. Asking more questions and gathering more information usually leads to more understanding and insight.

Emotions

Although emotions are aligned with the water element and the astral body, they arise from how sense data is recorded in the lower mind. If an activity is recorded as *liked*, emotions such as happiness, delight, or ecstasy arise. If an activity is recorded as *disliked*, emotions such as unhappiness, melancholy, gloominess, or despondency arise.

Emotions are often described as being like the weather – they come and go at a moment's notice. Sometimes they hang around for a while, but eventually, they give way to different conditions. The day may start with being cloudy and end with sunshine and rainbows. Emotions, like the weather, are temporary visitors. Emotions are neither inherently good nor inherently bad – they are simply information. It's what we do with our emotions and our reactions to them that needs investigation.

Using a camera analogy, we could think about emotions acting like a filter. Different filters can be applied to the camera lens using different settings; the settings adjust how the photographer wants to capture the environment, such as filtering how much light is included or excluded in the picture. The settings produce different results based on the photographer choosing which filters to use. The keyword is choice. We need to remember that we are choosing our reactions and, therefore, in a sense, emotions, albeit not always consciously.

We find some sage advice when we turn to sources such as the Yoga Sūtras of Patanjali and the Bhagavad Gita. Many students of Patanjali's Yoga Sūtras will be familiar with this aphorism: "yogaḥ citta vṛtti nirodhaḥ." I like to translate this aphorism as follows: *The path to inner freedom is the result of transcending the fluctuations of thoughts and feelings.* In this sutra, Patanjali points to a path of liberation and union, which can be experienced once the mind is stilled. Here, he is referring to the lower mind, which obscures both the true nature of all phenomena and the essence of the true Self. The mental modifications are all the forms in which the lower mind fabricates and obscures. It's not simply a matter of making the mind quiet, as in, you stop having thoughts. It's also not merely a matter of being able to observe your thoughts or mental content. One of the skills needed is harnessing the ability to disengage from thoughts once you're in them; next, disengage from thoughts as they arise, and then keep the mind clear. Disengaging from thoughts is a skill developed from neutrally observing the mind. Witnessing with emotional neutrality opens the door for drawing in the illumination of the higher mind. The light of the higher mind makes it possible to see and gradually dissolve the mental fabrications.

Although it's useful to think about cultivating the antidotes to mind states such as countering anger with love, the roots of that anger need to be weeded out. As a gardener, I can work relentlessly to pull up weeds that would choke out other important vegetation, but the weeds will continue to sprout up unless I get to the roots.

When the mind is caught up, as it were, in its projected experience of reality – liking or disliking something, judging something, an emotion arises. We become attached to something or someone. We cling or try to replicate experiences that we think made us happy. Or we become despondent or opposed to something or someone, pushing away what we think caused us pain. Liking or disliking becomes a repetitive cycle from which, as Patanjali suggests, we are liberated from when we can free ourselves from the habits of mind.

At various points throughout the conversation between Arjuna and Krishna, the Bhagavad Gita references liberation of the true Self by controlling the senses. In Chapter Two, for example, Krishna says to Arjuna: "When you keep thinking about sense objects, attachment comes. Attachment breeds desire, the lust of possession that burns to anger. Anger clouds the judgment; you can no longer learn from past mistakes. Lost is the power to choose between what is wise and what is unwise, and your life is utter waste. But when you move amidst the world of sense, free from attachment and aversion alike, there comes the peace in which all sorrows end, and you live in the wisdom of the Self" (Easwaran, E. p. 96).

Then in Chapter Three, Krishna says further: "The senses have been conditioned by attraction to the pleasant and aversion to the unpleasant. Do not be ruled by them; they are obstacles in your path" (Easwaran, E. p. 108).

One of the keys Krishna gives to Arjuna for bringing the senses under one's control is by cultivating non-attachment. At best, this can be described as a state of mind versus a skill. The essence of non-attachment is spiritual dispassion. Consciousness is unaffected by the senses. Personal will is aligned with the Universal will to create, learning and growth in service for the greater good of all beings. Non-attachment does not mean you don't have feelings or should not have feelings. It also does not suggest a feeling of apathy or ambivalence, which is very different from emotional neutrality and emotional calm. Non-attachment is not an extreme ascetic renunciation of the world; rather, it is a renunciation of all the fabrications of illusion that perpetuate the rebirth of saṃsāra. Waves may arise out of the ocean of experience, but they do not carry the wave-rider under the water. The wave-rider can stay on the wave, surfing as it were. Equanimity and non-attachment go hand in hand. As a state of mind, equanimity is an experience in which the inner observer is able to maintain a clear, calm presence while remaining undisturbed by the senses. In practice, the skill needed to cultivate this state of mind is where method and insight meet. The method is the form of exercises such as meditation or reflection. Insight opens to higher wisdom and deep intuitive knowing that penetrates and illuminates understanding. As these two meet, it becomes possible to dissolve obscurations, slowly wiping away dust from the mirror. (Refer to the practices at the end of the chapter for further guidance.) Gradually, deconstructing the fabricated self and realizing the true Self's nature makes it possible to free oneself inwardly from all self-imposed limitations.

As Krishna counsels Arjuna to follow his own dharma, he highlights the importance of living in alignment with one's own truth. Every step away from this alignment activates the senses becoming an additional source of suffering. "It is better to strive in one's own dharma than to succeed in the dharma of another. Nothing is ever lost in following one's own dharma, but competition in another's dharma breeds fear and insecurity" (Easwaran, E. p. 108). As with any belief or attitude, competition and insecurity are fabrications of the lower mind. The more skilled we become at witnessing the contents of our own mind and understanding their roots with higher wisdom, with the right tools, it becomes possible to gradually strip away the obscurations that hide the radiant beauty of the true Self.

Function of the Mind

A logical question to ask at this stage is: if the mind has all these ways of creating illusions, what then is the mind's purpose? To answer this question, we need to understand its role and function. Put simply, the role of the mind is a center of analysis. In its natural state, the mind makes no judgments about the information through which it's sorting. The natural state of the mind is neutral. Everything is regarded simply as information. In gathering and analyzing information, the mind expands or contracts depending on *what* is being processed.

We can think of this process as the aperture of a camera lens. Like the camera, the mind can focus on varying angles, such as a very wide angle to a very narrow angle of view. In a camera, the aperture controls how much the image is brought into focus, including how much light. Similarly, the mind changes the focus angle: zooming in for a more specific and detailed analysis or zooming out for a much larger scope of view. This zoom function can be dialed up or down, just like the camera's aperture. If the camera is not well-maintained, things like dust can build up on the lens. This build-up of dust can obscure the image.

On its own, a camera is just a camera. Once a photographer picks it up, the picture taker's job is to direct how the camera is used. The mind is not as "inert" as the camera sitting on a shelf gathering dust. But it is up to the person using the mind to direct it and use it appropriately. Herein lies the fundamental misunderstanding of the mind. Control is up to the user. If you buy a camera for the first time, you need to learn how to use it. There's the trial-and-error approach. You might read the manual first or read the manual alongside the camera, initiating functions as you go along. Or you might sign up for a class and receive some basic instruction as a new user, or more advanced instruction, the more comfortable and experienced you become with using the camera.

Without proper training, the mind can and does operate on its own. It can run wild, like an untrained horse. Unlike a camera that you can physically touch and see, it is more elusive to *see* the mind. It's not a physical, material thing. Mind-training with various exercises is like the camera user manual – you learn how to see the mind and operate the mind. One of the operations you bring under your control is the five senses. If you are sitting in a loud office and you need to concentrate, you may not realize the degree to which you're able to tune out most of the *noise*. Mind training takes this further. Mindfulness practices are another form of mind training, one of which teaches you how to turn your awareness inward. Mind training develops single-pointed focus, an essential skill not only for a more advanced meditation practice but also for using the mind as it is intended – an instrument of analysis.

Every individual has the power to liberate their mind. It is a courageous journey. Appropriate tools, skills, and support are necessary to harness this power. The reward, however, is immeasurable spiritual wealth, living in the joyful present.

Practice – Working with the mental fabrications

In this practice, the goal is to loosen up the mind where it's become tightly bound or rigid. Rigid thinking is generally rooted in having *likes* and *dislikes*, and it's useful to look at what they are to free oneself from self-imposed limitations. Gradually dissolving calcified *likes* and *dislikes* frees-up life force. It allows more light from the soul to shine through.

The practice begins with noticing whatever is part of your awareness without judgment. There is a difference between judgment and discernment. Judgment, in this context, takes a position that is polarized, i.e., like or dislike. In contrast, discernment uses common sense and wisdom to make choices and decisions. Judgment is rooted in the mental body, whereas discernment comes from the higher mind or causal body. Noticing without judgment enables one to recognize sense impressions as *information*. We then engage with curiosity to learn more about this information. We are looking for this in the practice – to initiate or re-initiate the learning process, curiosity being a fundamental component.

The first step is noticing without judgment. The second step is engaging with curiosity and examining reactions with wonderment. Curiosity opens up an inquiry, and a phrase that can be useful is something like, *that's interesting*. Questions to ask might be:

1. Is this automatic thinking running?
2. Why do I feel disappointed?
3. This reaction, such as disappointment, is an expectation; why?
4. What is it about this that I like?
5. What is it about this that I don't like?
6. What if I tried a different approach?

The more we're willing to consider strongly held likes and dislikes, it's possible to move categories of experience into a more flexible middle which can be thought of as *preferences*. Ultimately, the ideal is to find a balance where fewer likes and dislikes limit one's experience.

Practice – Working with emotions rooted in the mental body

Emotions develop and arise from thoughts first, not the other way around. Thoughts, such as obsessive thinking or judgments, will produce a general feeling that may or may not be perceptible to the ordinary waking consciousness. Eventually, feelings, when left unattended, give rise to an emotion. We learn to cultivate the opposite emotion to the one currently being experienced in the practice offered here. Therefore, the antidote is like medicine; the longer the treatment is applied, the more time it has to work through the system to heal the parts that need it. The practice does not specifically deal with *why* the emotion arose in the first place. While any emotion can be traced back to a thought or belief, the underlying cause and how to work with it is not the subject of this book.

The practice is intended to do two things. First, to awaken awareness in oneself and harness the power of the mind. Second, to move from feeling stuck to feeling and experiencing flow. We may not know *why* we are *angry*, but we can recognize that a more helpful emotion to cultivate is love, a more expansive and open-hearted emotion. Love amplifies your life force, raising your state of consciousness, filled with more of the light of the soul. A short list of emotions and possible antidotes are provided as a starting point in table 7.1.

The practice begins seated. Find a place to sit comfortably and relatively free of distractions. Settle into a meditation posture – chest open, arms relaxed, back upright, head slightly bowed toward the chest. As you close your eyes, establish a steady inward focus, slowing down the breath, syncing the mind with the breath. Effort should not be strained; rather, it should be gradual and steady. Establish a state of focus that is emotionally neutral – the witnessing state of consciousness. You can become aware of this as you recognize you are watching your breath and participating in the breath, such as adjusting the rhythm. From the state of emotional neutrality, bring to mind the challenging emotion.

Imagine the emotion typed out in letters. See these letters in your mind's eye, as if looking at them on a computer or TV screen. Imagine the letters of the word filling up with all your reactions and bodily sensations. Take your time with this step.

Once the letters are full, imagine burning them up until completely dissolved. The word is being burned up in the mental fire of illumination, which brings insight, wisdom, and inner peace. With this step complete, bring to mind the emotion opposite to the one just dissolved. Imagine the emotion typed out in letters. See these letters in your mind's eye, as if looking at them on a computer or TV screen. Imagine that these letters are filled with a radiant, joyful, and harmonious light. Imagine that light shining like rays of the sun and filling your mind. These rays stretch beyond the mind and now fill your heart center. Take your time with this step. After enough time has elapsed (which varies from person to person and practice session to practice session), shift your focus once again to the breath. Let the breath anchor you in the present moment and the body once more. Gradually open your eyes, returning to ordinary waking consciousness.

As with all other meditation practices offered in the book, use a journal to make any notes that feel important to record.

Table 7.1 – Emotions and antidotes

Negative Emotional State	Positive Emotional State
Anger	Love, patience, compassion, friendliness
Hate	Love
Envy	Empathic Joy
Ignorance	Open-ended inquiry that leads to wisdom
Fear	Open-ended inquiry
Desire/Attachment	Impermanence
Worry	Impermanence
Doubt	Patience and faith
Boredom/Procrastination	Open-ended inquiry
Resentment	Compassion
Ambivalence	Compassion and open-ended inquiry

Practice – Recognizing the impermanence in all things

All of life is in a constant state of change, with nothing ever truly permanent. The more we recognize and embrace the nature of impermanence, the more inner freedom is created. Embracing impermanence is often taught as a stage in some meditation and mind-training exercises. Each stage in the process lets in more light of higher illumination, which is the light of higher wisdom, insight, and the soul's perspective. The soul's perspective frees oneself from usual human tendencies at the root of much personal suffering.

We can see impermanence in all phenomena, beginning with our physical body. It's fairly uncommon to spend time noticing that the body is constantly changing. Yet it's plainly evident if you look at photos of yourself as a child next to photos of yourself as an adult. The body is constantly in cell growth, cell decline, cell death, and cell rebirth. If that were not the case, we would never grow and age. Recognizing the body's impermanence breaks down the attachment to the idea that it is permanent and unchanging.

If the body is impermanent, the natural next question involves feelings and emotions. We can think of emotions like the weather. Emotions come and go, like clouds passing through the sky. We might hold onto emotions as if they were permanent visitors, but even visitors eventually want to go home. Recognizing the impermanence of emotions breaks down the attachment to the idea that they are permanent and unchanging.

Similarly, thoughts are equally temporary. We may have some thoughts that are repeated, such as obsessively thinking about something. But even obsessive thinking is not as constant as the twenty-four-hour news cycle. More importantly, beliefs are not fixed statues of the mind. Beliefs shift and change as we grow and change. Many conflicts, both personal and the world, would benefit from a willingness to examine what new possibilities may be found if sclerotic beliefs could be changed. Recognizing the impermanence of thoughts and beliefs breaks down the attachment to the idea that they are permanent and unchanging. A very simplistic way to work with beliefs as changing is the practice of rearranging the furniture. Or less disruptive might be to move some photographs and paintings to new areas of the home. Think of this as a breaking down of seeing things the same way and refreshing one's perspective, knowing that the changes are not permanent. Even reading this book is an exercise in considering the possibility of new ideas and beliefs.

As we examine the changing nature of ourselves, we might also consider how we define those changes. As we've discussed in other sections of the book, each individual is more than a profession, job, title, or role. Today you might be working as a newspaper courier, and tomorrow you might be an entrepreneur of a new technology start-up. As we learn and grow, life constantly evolves and changes. Recognizing the impermanence of life provides an opening to the ever-evolving possibilities that surround us. You could say that the "great resignation" as a result of the global Covid-19 pandemic is the realization and discovery that many more possibilities exist than not.

Chapter 8

Fire

When we think of fire, most likely, the first image that comes to mind is something like a fire pit or a bonfire. Or if your fuel for cooking is wood, then perhaps it's the image of a wood-burning stove or open-aired fire. Fire is not only used as a source of fuel for cooking and heat for warmth. Fire is also alchemy, the power to transform, change, dissolve, and renew. A devastating forest fire will scorch everything in its path, causing mass destruction and chaos. Yet after the burn, new growth will emerge.

Fire has been used and honored by Indigenous cultures around the world for millennia. It was recognized early on for its power to create, heal, and destroy and great effort went into harnessing this power. In a traditional wood-fired pottery kiln, for example, an Anagama, functional pottery for everyday use can be made by utilizing the high heat of 2400º Celsius that the kiln generates. The melting point of steel which, at 2500ºF, will become a hot liquid, ready to be molded into a hard material. Fire is a transformational powerhouse. This transformational power is symbolized in spiritual terms as the power of purification, burning away all obscurations and illusions. Spiritual fire burns away all illusions so that the inner light of the transcendent Self may be visible.

Inner light is represented as another principle of the fire element, which is illumination. In material terms, we can relate to illumination as the ease of flipping on a light switch at home and having the lights turn on. But you may wonder, how does the light of the soul shine through? Think of it like an unobscured and open window that lets in sunlight on a clear day. Similarly, the soul's light can shine through when there are no obscurations, especially in the mind. When this light shines forth, the causal body represents the level of being from which each individual's life purpose exists. It exists in the form of energy and the radiance of the soul. More accurately, this energy is *dharma* which is the path that each person takes in their fulfillment of expressing who they are. Let's consider this as the degree to which there is enthusiasm and motivation for pursuing the fulfillment of one's dharma, as well as all other areas of life that increase satisfaction and joy. Fire then represents the extent to which *individual dharma* is being expressed, no matter the form. *Dharma* is a Sanskrit word that does not have a distinct English equivalent. It can be understood to mean the "way," or "a path," that unfolds as the soul plan for each individual. As is natural with the way languages evolve, dharma has found its way into more common usage in the West, mixing this original Sanskrit word with English vocabulary. However, dharma is usually equated with a more narrow definition as "life purpose," where life purpose is associated with a profession or a career. Even though an assigned or adopted label may be limited, it still serves the function of identification.

Identity is the agglomeration of labels that are useful for orienting toward something or away from something. For example, a person may choose to be an architect instead of a craftsperson of fine cabinet making. The forms are different but related – they share an underlying energy to express a creative principle of making forms. I've noticed more recently that the term "maker" is being used by craftspeople of varying styles and traditions, in addition to describing their work as "furniture maker" or "quilter," for example. The term "maker" is apt. It represents the underlying essence, where the term "furniture maker" is a distinct label. Suppose I need a table – I know that I need to look for a furniture maker.

Each person has their own unique identity, a non-physical container made up of multitudinous components, serving the function of expressing the soul into physical reality. The fire of illumination shines a light on seeing the essence of an individual (the composition of fire) rather than seeing them as the outwardly defined identity (the visible flames). While this is a chapter about the fire element, Bruce Lee's advice that draws on the water element is nevertheless relevant when he says, "be like water; water has form and yet it has no form," the analogy of which describes the experience of form and formlessness (Lee. p. 108). The same analogy can be applied to the fire element. Fire at this level is the burning away of the illusions that confuse identity as being a real independent reality rather than what is the true reality, the transcendent Self, which is beyond form. If we think of dharma as an evolution, or "the law of the next stage of its unfolding," it is inherently, formless (Besant, A. p. 12).

The second significant component of the principle of illumination is wisdom. Wisdom is not a measure of a person's IQ (intelligence quotient). Wisdom is the depth of insight and knowing, and it illuminates every level of being, especially the mind. Whenever we can shine a light on something previously hidden or obscured in some way, it is often accompanied by an experience of total clarity. The hottest part of a flame is when a white edge surrounds a translucent center of the flame. We can, therefore, think of this as the inner wisdom and illumination burning cleanly and brightly.

A fire that burns too hot risks burning everything around it, even extinguishing itself when nothing is left to combust. On the other hand, there is insufficient energy to power something like a stove for heat or cooking if there is too little fire. The energy of personal power and living fully from one's own dharma is fueled with an ever-burning fire of passion, creativity, and a willingness to experiment. All creativity is a symbolic expression of some form of fire. Learning is and of itself a creative process filled with experimentation along the way. The experiments may be messy at times, and sometimes they work out just as you had planned or imagined. The important thing to remember is that the lesson is more important than getting something *right* or *perfect*. Perfectionism is too much fire, burning so hot that everything in its path, including the fire itself, is burned up in its blinding blaze. Instead, a balanced fire element reminds us to come back to the middle and play. At the heart of playfulness is the joy of being in the moment and the experience, enjoying the process at hand, and having fun. The spiritual path need not be serious all the time.

Expression

As stated before, everyone has a unique path and a specific set of lessons that they are learning. However, it is important to realize that a path does not mean that there is only one way to express oneself and the core of one's being. Expression of all the varied interests a person may have is just as important as expressing and living from one's dharma. One way to think about these interests is hobbies such as knitting or needlepoint or other forms of crafting. A person might knit scarves and blankets for themselves, their friends, or their family. The hobby or activity is a satisfying experience from the moment the pattern for a new scarf is conjured, who it might be for, to then giving it to the person as a surprise gift. Hobbies are not the only way to express the many interests and pursuits a person may enjoy, and they aren't necessarily about how one earns a living. A person might be an avid cyclist, partaking in specially planned bike trips with a cycling group. Gardening is another, using as many spare moments to plant, prune and harvest. Together with dharma, whatever the hobbies and avid interests are, they form the multidimensional picture of expressing who an individual is, radiating and shining all their beauty into the world.

Connection

At this point, we have connected with a person physically, emotionally, and mentally. Now, we open ourselves to connecting with them at the deepest level, the soul. The soul is more than the ego-personality of a person, which itself is a veil. As we've stated before, the soul is an energy, an essence. Connection at this level is from one soul to another, seeing one another at the very core of each other's being. This core of the soul, as an expression of the Source, is divine. The most fundamental of all human needs is to be seen, heard, and understood. At this level, it is the most profound need of all to be met in this way. As someone might invite a friend or a stranger to their home, connecting at the soul level is an invitation for them to come home to their true Self and see that in each other. We may find this depth of connection with a family member, a close friend, a life partner, a group. The groups of relationships form a circle of spiritual community – safely sharing the deepest level of the Self.

Alignment

The soul is always speaking, inviting us to live from the truth of who we are. To hear the soul speak means to listen deeply and inwardly. There is always guidance from within, and it takes patience, practice, and persistence to allow that guidance to light the way forward. Sometimes it takes courage to follow one's dharma, whether that means tuning out the inner voice that says "it's impossible or unachievable" or the outside voices that would say the same. Each person is tasked with two things: living from their true Self and sharing this truth with the world. The more each person lives in alignment with their unique dharma, the greater this benefits us all, including oneself. Alignment with the true Self is, in essence, to be in alignment with the Universe.

Summary – Skill in Action

To embody a balanced fire element is to live from the experience of flow-based reality creation. Working with the Universe's flow, including all sentient beings, an individual is in touch, directly or indirectly, with a cooperative attitude that values participation. The Universe is based on a principle of interdependence. To live in recognition and alignment with this principle means to realize that the more one lives from their unique dharma, the more this benefits the web of shared interconnection. More positive energy flows in and around oneself. Life is once again, as it always was, experienced as magical.

Practice – Interdependence

A universal principle applicable to all of us is that we live in a causal Universe. It is also true that we live in a universe that is inherently and fundamentally interdependent. The food available for purchase on the grocery store shelves did not arrive there by chance, luck, or a wish. Someone had to do something to grow that food, package it, ship it, and stock it on the shelf. Universally, when life seems to *go our way*, most if not all of us experience a sense of delight and joy that life has unfolded so seamlessly. It can be small moments, like when the traffic lights are all green for both directions of the work commute, or larger moments, like when a long trip with many flights flowed without any cancelations or delays. We can choose to think of those moments as *chance*, or we can choose to see those moments as the incredible mechanics of a system working together in harmony. This harmony is flow-based living, and it is a joyous and satisfying experience from which to live. The practice begins with attuning one's awareness to the orchestra of interdependence, noticing all the moments when a harmonious balance has been created, and you are one part of that balance. It can begin in the routine daily movements, making toast for breakfast, or brewing coffee. We can think about the fact that other people were involved in producing these items. Let's think more deeply about the production chain of the coffee in this scenario:

- Who was involved in preparing the soil, harvesting the beans, roasting the beans, and packaging the beans?
- How was the planet affected in producing the coffee beans? Has the soil been over-harvested to the point of depletion?
- How were the beans transported? Who was involved in the transportation chain?

I think you get the idea. The next step involves a choice. It is a choice to either be a willing participant and co-creator benefiting oneself and others or not. Choosing to be a co-creator shifts one's awareness about the process but also the values and attitudes we would like to hold about ourselves and the world. Flow or a state of flow is like a magical stream that carries everything within it in perfect balance and harmony. We can align with this flow or not. We can either flow *with the river* or try to *push the river*. Once we are aligned with flow, the last step in completing our understanding and alignment of interdependence is gratitude. Gratitude is being thankful for the support received in being carried, uplifted, and guided in such a way that every step flowed effortlessly. Cultivating gratitude is good preparation for developing heart-centered and unity consciousness, a hopeful next step in the evolution for all of humanity.

Practice – Inner Guidance

Everyone has within themselves an inner teacher, a Self-generated navigation and guidance system. At any given moment, this navigation system may be unavailable to one's awareness and waking consciousness. As with an electrically powered navigation system that needs fuel to operate, we can similarly think of the internal combustion of individual navigation. Internal combustion is the fire element, and sometimes, it needs to be reignited. Re-ignition is an awakening to inner Self-trust, listening inwardly to inner guidance, stepping into one's personal power, and giving oneself permission to live from and inhabit one's dharma.

Two mutually dependent components align oneself with this level of being and state of consciousness. The first component is the desire and willingness to enter into this inner conversation. In a sense, it's an invitation for the self as personality to meet the Self as soul at their intersecting boundary. Invitations by their nature are a sign of being welcomed. Whenever we feel genuinely welcomed, we may naturally feel inwardly safe enough to expand our boundaries, allowing the vulnerability of opening those boundaries to bring us closer together. The second component involves inner stillness. Mental equipoise, which is developed in the earlier stages, sets the foundation for the soul's voice to be heard. Imagine going to a library, a place marked by a search for knowledge within an atmosphere of quiet seeking.

In contrast, imagine a lively bookstore with an attached café filled with the cacophony of whirring coffee machines buzzing over both hushed and vibrant conversations. Mental equipoise is more like the quiet seeking of the library versus the cacophonous café. The inner atmosphere that is serene, steady, and quietly seeking without urgency but rather genuine curiosity opens the channel for the soul's voice to be heard.

I've recommended the use of a journal in earlier sections of the book. The process of writing down one's thoughts continues to be one of the most useful methods in developing a personal daily spiritual practice, which simply means, a practice of becoming closer to and more intimate with knowing oneself more deeply. The journal simply acts as the medium. One way to think about using the journal here is to ask for guidance. A blank page is opened in the journal, and a question or request is written at the top of the page such as, *What is the appropriate next step I need to take?* or *I am in need of inner guidance, please help.* Notice the way in which the question and request are phrased. Both are open-ended, neither of them is demanding nor urgent, no willfulness is involved. This is important as it frees the writing, and thus the dialogue, between the self as personality and the Self as soul to be open and transparent without the interference of the usual ways the lower mind gets caught up in polarized thinking. The writing may feel a bit clunky and awkward to start with, but as the process unfolds so does a sense of flow and ease with the words naturally becoming etched on the page. In other words, thinking and time momentarily pause. When the writing comes to a natural conclusion, then it's time to review what was written. Try this out every day for a few months. It may become a regular part of one's daily spiritual practice.

Chapter 9

Karma

The word karma is originally a Sanskrit term, but it has made its way into our common everyday language, in particular, here in the West. I often hear the word used casually as someone having "earned good karma" or someone "deserving what they got because of bad karma." This is a very simplistic view, missing a lot more of the nuance of what it means and one that I believe can lead to actually creating more karma instead of less. It's important to clear up a few misunderstandings of what karma is not. Karma is not the result of either a *good* action or a bad action. Actions themselves are neither rewarded nor punished. Karma is also not predetermined, nor unchangeable, nor destiny. Very importantly, it is not something that you have no control over. It is not about "luck," whether you have it or don't have it, nor if it's good or bad. Now that we've explained what karma isn't let's talk about what karma is.

A basic definition of karma is this – it is a universal principle based upon a causal relationship. Using the analogy of an apple tree, we can demonstrate this principle as it unfolds. The causal chain begins with a **seed (thought)** like the seed of an apple **(form)**. This seed is full of **potential**, holding within itself the possibility to **create** a new tree **(manifested form)**. It may or may not **germinate** if the conditions required are not present. Not all the seeds from fallen fruit produce new **trees (dormant)**. When a seed does take root, all the potential that was dormant now begins to **ripen**. A tree is born **(result)**.

You may wonder, why bother understanding what karma is? It's simple, really. To liberate oneself from dissatisfaction, unhappiness, and suffering is to take responsibility for the world a person themselves creates. This happens not outside oneself but inside, in one's own mind and heart. Although karma and mind are treated as separate chapters in the book, they are, in fact, inexorably linked. However, it can be easier for us to conceptualize these principles by drawing them out separately and then slowly working through them little by little.

Karma is also dealt with under the meta-view of the element of fire for two reasons. First, fire is the light of illumination, wisdom, and higher knowledge or insight. Karma, in a sense, is a vehicle for teaching a path out of illusion and bondage (the ego) to the higher perspective of the lesson and, ultimately, inner freedom (the soul). Second, fire represents the causal body, the radiance of the true Self shining through into physical reality, exploring and experiencing the form of materiality. But that radiance can be blocked from shining for many reasons, and one way to understand those blockages is to understand the associated karma.

In the iconography that depicts the wheel of rebirth or samsara, one of its lessons is that freedom from this seemingly endless repetitive cycle is awakening. "Shakyamuni Buddha, for example, referred to this condition (the circle of perpetual frustration) of repeated dissatisfaction as samsara – a Sanskrit term meaning 'to circle,' – and prescribed many different methods for liberating ourselves from it" (Lama Yeshe. p. 20). This awakening is the process of burning away all illusions (fire that dissolves) and allowing the light of wisdom and insight (fire of illumination) to guide your path. This path requires effort and serious dedication. There are no shortcuts.

So, how do we effectively deal with karma? We start with examining the causal chain, and in the process, cultivate the skills to recognize where change is needed in order to draw ourselves closer to shining our inner radiance out into the world. The causal chain of karma and reincarnation is discussed in the Brihadaranyaka Upanishad. As stated at the beginning of Chapter Seven, this early Upanishad offers the view that *your thoughts become your words. From your words, you develop your actions. From your actions you create your reality.* Right from the start, this short aphorism points to the mind as the beginning. From thoughts, physical reality manifests. **Your thoughts create your reality.** Everything begins in the mind, whether it is a desire for a new house or new job, finding a love relationship, and discovering your life purpose. In the mind, the wheel is set into motion. Along the way, internal and external forces are marshaled to help bring this intention into physically manifested form. Like a wheel in perpetual motion, life keeps turning as it's propelled by the forces of satisfaction and dissatisfaction, likes and dislikes. Usually, when we complain about having an experience that is unpleasant, not liking something, the usual human reaction is to blame – that some external force created it. We can't possibly imagine that we ourselves were at the very beginning of generating the experience. The choices we make every day, including not choosing or believing that no choice exists, are rooted in the mind and based on our beliefs and values. These beliefs and values shape our worldview and how we act within the world. We are always making choices, and as such, the responsibility for those choices rests within us.

As with the apple seed in our earlier analogy, intentions and thoughts need a vehicle to express themselves in a physical form, similar to the apple tree. The vehicle is what is called a *samskara*. I like to think of a samskara as a container. The container fills up, like a bottle, with thoughts and feelings amassed over some period of time. It could be days, it could be weeks, or it could be months. Now, imagine the bottle is filled with soda, and is sealed under pressure. If you've ever had the experience of opening a soda bottle that was violently shaken, you'll recall the explosiveness of the liquid inside that suddenly pours out in every direction. A samskara that is ready to empty out is like a bottle under a pressure that is suddenly released, and often, with surprising and unexpected consequences. It's important to note that a samskara is created even if the intentions are unconscious. We are, therefore, once more called back to the mind, for it is here where obscurations and illusions need to be brought into full view in order for them to be changed or dissolved. And it is here where we draw in the light of higher wisdom, insight, discernment, and illumination. In practice, this is something that is cultivated gradually over a long period of time.

Karma – step by step

Working with karma involves a multi-step process. We examine not only the consequences of our actions in the present, but also the impact it could have in the future. From a multi-life point of view, karma travels with us from one lifetime to the next. *Samskaras* can influence how a lifetime unfolds, and although it is possible to access a past life, it's not specifically necessary. One way I've come to think about past life karma is that for some of my experiences that have no reasonable present lifetime origin, I attribute those experiences to a carry-over. Thinking in this way expands my ability to generate greater self-compassion toward myself, and hence to others. Therefore, regardless of whether or not we have insight into a prior lifetime, we most definitely have the power to examine our own hearts and mind right here, in the present moment.

The first step is to recognize that you're dissatisfied with something. Possibly too, you recognize a pattern that keeps repeating itself, a cycle which you can't seem to break. You are ready for change, are motivated to break the cycle. This stage could be called **motivated awareness**; you need to want change and be willing to do the work. Change will not happen if you simply wish for it.

With motivated awareness, it's now possible to begin the examination of the causes of the current distress. As has been stated, reality is manifested first from thought and then through action. This stage could be called **investigation**; we examine the seeds that generate the results of experience, some of which operate as deep-seated blindspots. It should be kept in mind that this stage is not fast. There can be no self-imposed or other imposed timeline for how long it takes to reach a deep understanding of some of life's larger lessons.

All experiences result from a process of learning, which in turn develops into growth. This process is fueled by a) the will to create and b) the desire to experience. Neither of these two impulses is inherently bad nor good. They are simply an energy that propels experience. The real stickiness arises with thinking how and what that should or should not be. The basic categories that create stickiness broadly fall under clinging and aversion. [A large subject which is only briefly touched upon further in the chapter on mind.]

It would be inaccurate to assume that simply "not wanting" or "just getting over things" or somehow getting rid of "attachment" will bring about lasting change. Step-by-step, you examine the source of the particular form of clinging and aversion which you're examining. It means examining the core beliefs and attitudes that essentially shape your perception of reality and how you create it. This is where the role of mentors, teachers, guides, partners, trusted friends are essential. Some traditions emphasize the need for studying in pairs. This is because there is an innate understanding that we all need a reflection, lest we become stuck in our own echo chamber.

Ideally, understanding karma, your own and others, is the recognition that every event is a lesson. The forces of karma are always looking for optimal conditions for growth; once we see the lesson as a gift, we will have realized our fundamental truth. Karma operates for the greater good of all, which strives for balance and harmony.

Chapter 10

Space

Space is all around us. It's in and around physical objects. It's between ourselves and others. There is space between the body's internal organs. Space is in and around all of Nature. Space is an all-pervading element from which all the other elements arise, is boundless and boundary-less. A perhaps common misperception is thinking that air and the atmosphere are space since air is usually not detectable with our ordinary visual perception. As the pervasive and all-penetrating element, the underlying principle of space is a unifying force, drawing us back to our essential unity with all others and our essential unity with the Source of all Being.

Unlike the other four elements, space is a vast unlimited emptiness. Perhaps another way to think about emptiness is that it is voidness. Conceptually, it can be difficult for the mind to conceive of emptiness and voidness. Naturally, we might want to think of the void as *nothingness*. However, nothingness implies annihilation. An erroneous view, annihilation, suggests a total extinguishment of the existence of anything. Space, or the void, is a formless state. It is a primordial state of matter. Phenomena arise out of this state and dissolve back into this state. It is naturally radiant, brighter than the sun.

As we attempt to conceive of space, our task is to realize that we are in a steady state of flux, moving into form and moving out of form. What does this mean? Form, such as the body, is the container for an experience. All forms are temporary, including their identity, and exist for some length of time. Time, therefore, represents an arc of learning and growth experience. Once the form has reached its point of usefulness, it undergoes a process of dissolution back into the state from which it arose, which is the void. All experiences are integrated within the formless state.

The process of dying, death, and rebirth is one such process of moving into and out of form. The habitual attachment to the physical body, a person's identity, and a fear of death contribute to a sticky process of moving into and out of form. There is a belief that everything material, including the body, is real and unchanging; even a person's identity or personality is perceived as itself being a material and permanent form. However, the unlimited Self does not die; rather, it transforms each time it sheds the container of a physical body.

I'll use an analogy that will be familiar to most people. A typical progression for a child receiving an education is going through the various school stages, from kindergarten to high school. Within each year, a series of semesters or terms cover different subjects. As the semester progresses, each class goes deeper, expanding on the material to be learned. At the end of a semester, two things usually occur. Typically, tests or exams assess students' memory, understanding, and comprehension of the material learned. Second, there is a school break, as short as one week or as long as one month. The break period is an essential component of the learning process for the individual to integrate and assimilate everything that has been learned. Integration is a vitally important stage in any area of learning. The school term represents the form, and the break represents the dissolution of the form, even if only temporarily. Learning does not end when an individual graduates from high school. Learning continues – only the form itself changes.

The process of moving into and out of the formless state, space, is an essential component of transformation. A caterpillar that spins its cocoon becomes a butterfly. Human beings regularly shed an old Self to become a new Self. Consider how a person might describe the experience of themselves after, for example, a vacation. You might hear them say in jubilance: *wow,*

I feel like a new person! Or, a person that undertook a months-long pilgrimage might say: *the experience completely transformed me!* Of course, one doesn't have to undertake a pilgrimage to shed an old self! Rather, an awareness is developed wherein a person recognizes that this is a natural part of a lifetime cycle, day-to-day, week-to-week, month-to-month, year-to-year.

When a person experiences a state of voidness, even if it is only a brief glimpse, it can feel like an ultimate bliss. The bliss state, as it is sometimes referred to in various teachings of yoga, is not an end state in and of itself. Rather, the liberation of moksha points to only one state out of many possibilities. In the experience of *a* bliss state, the boundaries of the false self temporarily dissolve, making it possible to merge with the space-like void.

A word of caution. Even for experienced meditators, preparation and foundation are essential, including the support of an experienced guide or teacher. Insufficient stability within one's core Self makes this transition into and out of void-like states challenging for the personality because there is an inherent fear of being annihilated and dissolved into nothingness. Entering and returning from void states is not something to be rushed by anyone, in oneself, or anyone else. Without proper understanding, spiritual maturity, and sufficient mental stability, the lines may start to blur, making the distinction between what is real and what is false difficult to discern.

I have often thought that the ego-personality construct has largely been misunderstood as something that can be dispensed with, thus erasing its influence. In my mind, this reflects a fundamental misunderstanding of its role; it is not meant to be in the director's seat. Rather, it is intended to take direction from a higher authority, the soul. A result of this misunderstanding is an internal battle of will for dominance because the ego-personality fears that it will die.

Resolving this internal battle requires understanding the nature of the evolution of a soul's growth. The soul gradually and organically unfolds itself, dissolving illusions and obscurations to live more and more from its true nature. Clinging to selfishness is slowly stripped away, another form of falsely perceiving separateness. In the process, the core Self stabilizes, and the ego-personality becomes integrated, like a chariot for its rider. Thus, the door opens to a state of union, the primordial state from which we never were separated and which the unlimited Self first emerged upon its individuation from the Source.

The natural outcome of being merged within the union state is called joy. Joy is a natural state of radiant balance, not to be confused with happiness which is an emotion. Joy naturally expresses itself in the moment wherein all four elements have come together in a state of ideal balance, held together within the tender embrace of the fifth element, space. As a point of comparison, when a single or all elements are out of balance, we have dropped out of the state of joy. In the unmanifest state, all four elements exist in their unlimited potential, held in a dynamic stillness. The unmanifest state, holding all unlimited potential in perfect equilibrium, is a naturally radiant and joyful state of consciousness. Joy is, therefore, always present, and always available. As we find greater alignment with ourselves, with others, with Nature, and with the Universe itself, the possibility of living from joy is ever-present. Self-liberation is essentially a process of freeing oneself from the habit of being form-bound. When that habit dissolves, consciousness is able to focus more and more on living from joy in the present moment.

Turning awareness from moment to moment, staying in the present, and a willingness to experiment with all the unlimited possibilities that life offers are necessary for becoming more attuned to the element of space. In addition, there are particular principles that, once familiar with, can help turn awareness in their direction, which can essentially be called *unity consciousness*. These principles are:

1. Fundamentally, all life is interdependent.
2. The Universe is nourished with unlimited Grace.
3. Harmony and Balance are indivisible.

Unity consciousness, which is the near constant embodied realization of the oneness with all things, can also be called *heart consciousness*. In our framework of the five elements, the Sanskrit word for space is *ākāśa*, the subtle atmosphere or ether that permeates through the Universe. However, its second meanings of *radiance* is the result of a later development wherein the seat of consciousness of the true Self was thought to reside in the heart center. The way I think about the energy of the Source is that it's a radiant, effulgent glow, brighter than the sun. Each individual, containing a microcosm of the Source, therefore holds this radiant energy and light with them, which we can connect with by reaching into heart consciousness (Feuerstein, Georg. p. 17).

The more we become ourselves, namely the core Self, and strip away the fear of separation and division, the closer we come to a greater Universal union. Heart consciousness, the next chapter, guides us toward this ideal as we examine the specific values and intentions that shape our trajectory.

Working with integration

One way to think about working with integration is to recognize it as a stage in the process of learning and growth. Every stage is a culmination of events shaping the overall arc of the soul's journey in a lifetime, whether it's the ups and downs of a single day, selling a home, starting a new business, or ending a relationship. Often unrecognized if not underappreciated, the integration phase is generally rushed through if not skipped entirely, even though it's a vital component of any learning and growth process.

I was on a personal quest to learn to bake bread. This quest happened to coincide with a bread baking craze that symbolized the unfolding global Covid-19 pandemic in the year 2020. I started with what appeared to be a fairly straightforward recipe. I followed all the steps, at least I thought I had. And I watched some video tutorials. But alas, I had yet to produce something edible. Fortunately, a very dear friend offered to teach me how to make a loaf of bread. Through the process of transmitting his experience, including some fundamentals that I had missed, together we baked some delicious homemade bread! There was a moment in which I realized what I had accomplished, followed by the feeling of personal celebration, fulfillment, and satisfaction. I wanted to savor the moment — like the aroma of fresh baking, to breathe in the joy of the moment. Each slice eaten over the next few days provided another moment to savor and reflect on the experience. In a way, eating the bread became a literal symbol of integrating the learning experience.

There are three signals to the process to pay attention to:

1. Basking in joy
2. Reflecting on learning
3. Slowing down

The first signal is, as it says – basking in joy. It's stopping long enough in the moment to savor the joy and satisfaction from the learning experience. As our example above illustrates, this may include reflecting on the joy and gratitude of spending time with a dear friend. In the second signal, we reflect on what we learned, such as gaining new skills. It may also reflect the value of patience in the learning process where there had been a tendency to rush or quit. With the third signal, slowing down smooths out the integration process so that it may be completed.

Anytime there is a desire to rush the process before completing the preceding step, the vital stage of integration is skipped. Think about the steps involved in the following situations and what each stage might look like:

1. Buying a new house in a new neighborhood
2. Moving to a new city or new country
3. Changing a profession to something completely new
4. Starting a new job in a new town or new country
5. Going on a first date after a long-term relationship of five years has ended

Integration offers us a juncture to dive into the liminal space between beginnings and endings. We can tap into this space whether we're following a self-guided journey or being facilitated by someone else such as a therapist, coach, mentor, spiritual counselor, or trusted friend.

Going deeper

The five elements offer a template for reading the energy of a space, room, and or group and the skillful methods for affecting useful and meaningful change. By tapping into your intuitive inner sense perceptions, it's possible to draw a mental image of all the non-verbal information that is available and present in the moment. As a facilitator, this can be an invaluable aid in delivering the message effectively while being responsive to the dynamics of the energies interacting with one another. Walking into a room full of people may not necessarily be a positive, jovial experience. Strangers united by a common interest may all be sitting quietly, perhaps a little nervous as they wait for the presenter. A facilitator recognizes the group needs an ice-breaker to move energy and draws upon the air element to inject a sense of humor and lightness into the dynamic. The facilitator, this example, illustrates the potential for positive change in their ability to recognize and read the energy in the group. The skill of reading energy is not unique to someone specially trained. Every human being is capable of perceiving the energy of others. The skill lies in how much greater our capacities are for meeting the moment with more awareness and compassion.

This section starts by asking a series of questions that can be considered in different circumstances. We then offer a sample of possibilities for balancing energies based on what is discovered. As a suggestion, try to think of three or four different situations that provide a selection from which it's possible to draw comparisons of the different ways the energies of the elements show up. In general, this type of practice can be applied in all areas of life.

Subtle element questions:

1. How does/did the overall balance of elements (earth, water, air, fire, space) feel in the room?
2. Which element seemed to be most out of balance in the individual/group?
3. What factors could have been influencing the energy of the group? (For example, local, national, or international events.)
4. Was this a new situation or a new group, people previously unknown to you, or was there some familiarity? (Your element(s) interacting with the elements of the other students, and they then interact with you and each other.)
5. What noticeable shifts were evident from the time the class/event/meeting began to when it ended?
6. What did you notice about yourself and how your energy shifted?

Subtle element possibilities:

1. If the room felt lively, cheerful, and upbeat, this would reflect the enthusiasm and passion of the fire element.

Conversely, if it felt cold, withdrawn, and eerily quiet, this would reflect the distant and impersonal nature of the air element.

2. Inviting the individual or group into a practice of conscious breathing utilizes the grounding energy of the earth element to draw air back into the body, i.e., embodied consciousness. Similarly, using the same practice can soften and focus the eager energy of fire, i.e., embodied concentration.

3. The flux of energies for an individual or group, including oneself, is influenced moment to moment. Personal events, local community situations, and national and even international events can directly or indirectly influence the balance of the subtle elements affected.

4. In a situation where you don't know the group or the information being presented is new, there may be a tendency to default to a less comfortable element. Freezing up (water) and not feeling grounded (earth).

5. Shifting energies reflect how much the elements came into balance together, resulting in feelings of cohesiveness, symmetry, and overall balance.

6. If you arrived feeling a little ungrounded and disembodied (not enough earth) throughout the presentation, this might have shifted to feeling more calm, steady, and at ease (i.e., balanced earth).

This next section offers a series of prompts that may be considered when structuring a class, presentation, workshop, meeting, or consultative session.

1. How might a class or workshop be arranged or structured around the focus of a particular element?

2. A survey can be useful for gathering information in situ, which might be as simple as "how are/is you/everyone

feeling?" The response(s) can inform what mix of energies may be in play.

3. In the situation of facilitating an individual (coaching, mentoring, guidance, healing, etc.), how can you best support them in: restoring balance with a particular element, or shedding light on a blindspot, or responding to a specific need?

4. What specific practices may be useful? For example, a breathing practice that reestablishes a connection to the body.

In asking questions and examining information from the particular viewpoint of the five elements, the possibility of awakening the intuitive inner sense perceptions increases. A wealth of non-physical information is always available to us for insight, healing, learning, and growth. Every individual has the capacity to awaken to these inner non-physical dimensions. It begins with focusing questions and curiosity in this direction. Becoming more fully developed compassionate and empathic human beings is not just a possibility. It is a necessary step if we are to collectively move in the direction of harmonious union with all of life. Small steps have an incremental and cumulative benefit over time, one day at a time.

Going deeper

Attunement is a process of bringing oneself into harmony, in this case, with a set of ideals and principles. Attunement is applied using a short statement repeated a few times inwardly at first, then revisited periodically over time. In a sense, this is like downloading a template into the energetic field of your own operating system. The template functions to draw yourself into closer alignment and harmony with the intention. It works outwardly to draw to yourself all the resources and support in similar alignment with the intention. Whenever there is greater alignment with the core Self, there is usually an accompanying increase in the flow of life force. More life force is associated with the experience of increasing satisfaction and an expression of joy. The practice of using an energetic template thus works to bring oneself into harmony and alignment with an ideal as well as to bring one back into balance with it. Therefore, this practice works with two subjects covered in the book: balancing and harmonizing with the five elements and harmonizing and living from the universal values of harmony. Attunement works through the agency of intention to bring about some change within oneself.

To begin with, I recommend first reading through the list. This first step should provide a sense of the levels at which the statements are working. It will also guide you to feel into where you might need to begin. In general, the practice is not intended to be followed in sequential order, nor is it meant to be prescriptive. Instead, use your intuition and listen inwardly as you feel into the words. Pay attention to feelings that arise, such as ambivalence, aversion, interest, or attraction. Read slowly, allowing the energy of the words to sink in. Try to pause for a moment before reading the next statement. As an ongoing practice, you could perhaps write out the full list or one particular statement and place it somewhere in your home that's used for contemplation or meditation, such as an altar.

Another way to work with the attunements is to begin reading through each one and pause for ten seconds. The next step might be daily, such as for seven days. After seven days, the process of reading and reflecting could be repeated once a week for three weeks, then repeated monthly for three months, and adding thirty minutes of contemplative journaling. The journaling is focused on your own assessment of noticing changes in your thoughts, words, actions, and interactions due to the choice to align yourself with these principles.

For instance, as a longer-term practice over a further nine months, the attunements could be revisited once a quarter with a continued regular journaling practice.

The ending of a calendar year offers a valuable opportunity to reflect on the past, reviewing and taking inventory of areas of learning and growth. A year-end reflection could be incorporated, reflecting on how these attunements may have influenced changes in yourself, your life, and those around you. As an ongoing practice, revisit the list as you feel inward guidance or whenever there is a feeling of misalignment.

The first four attunements are more general while the remaining four deal specifically with the four elements.

The attunements (included here with permission) of *non-violence* [2011–2022], *truth* [2011–2022], *earth* [2014], *water* [2014], *air* [2014], and *fire* [2014], are drawn from handwritten transcriptions of oral teachings I have received from my spiritual studies with Kurt Leland.

Non-Violence

One of the many values of this practice is how it guides you toward living from non-harmfulness moment to moment.

Attunement: I am responsible for my actions and reactions, none of which are intended to harm another.

Effort

Annie Besant says that "effort which has ignorance behind it, however well-intentioned it be, does more harm than good." In other words, we still create karma or the result of actions out of ignorance.

Attunement: Right effort and action guided by right knowledge.

Truth

No truth is absolute. Everyone has their own truth which can be thought of as their unique path in life, or dharma.

Attunement: Truth that guides without judgment.

Surrender

There is a higher power that runs through the Universe. As stated earlier in the book, this we refer to as the Source. A willingness to align with and open to a higher universal will from the Source, opens the self-boundary to the flow of grace.

Attunement: I surrender to the grace and love of the Source of All Being.

Earth element

Attunement – for groundedness and standing in the center of my world.

Water element

Attunement – for flow and the ability to adapt to every condition.

Air element

Attunement – for clarity and the ability to take the next step.

Fire element

Attunement – for motivation and the ability to burn through all illusions and obstacles.

Chapter 11

Balancing the Elements

The challenge with any practice and life itself is to strike the balance of discovering and living from the middle way. This means that we are always being called back to a state of being that is operating in the center rather than from an extreme on one side or another. We see this fundamental principle working all around us when we look to Nature which maintains a delicate balance across the entire planet while constantly moving.

With a foundation in place for the five elements, the next step is developing a practice for working with them, bringing them into balance, maintaining that balance, and integrating their lessons. Working with the elements can be viewed as a form of spiritual practice. It has daily application without opposition to other traditions that may already form part of an existing spiritual belief system. **Spiritual practice at its heart is the path that brings an individual closer to their own soul and closer to the Source of All Being.**

Moving through the practices, I encourage you to notice several things, including:

- how you feel
- where or how your levels of self-understanding change
- areas of particular challenge as you self-remember
- when you feel a greater sense of inner peace
- changes in your inner dialogue
- the moments when you feel a sense of joy
- changes in your relationships
- how you feel in your body
- the feeling of increasing life force and vitality

- the moments when everything is in a state of flow and ideal harmony.

Noticing these changes helps orient your consciousness toward rather than away from greater flow, balance, and harmony.

Orientation

Every individual is a composition and balance of the elements. The first relationship we identify is which element expresses itself within us most prominently. The more prominently expressed element is the one that principally shapes the way we create our own reality, the one we usually draw upon first. Although it's the element that may be the "easiest" to work with, it can and does go out of balance. The function of ranking the elements in order from most easy to most difficult serves to understand better our blindspots. It also highlights areas that are of a greater or lesser challenge. It's then possible to create balance and experience integration.

Relationship dynamics are formulated and affected by the interaction of the elements as expressed in each person. Therefore, a useful tool in navigating the ups and downs of relationships is understanding the interaction of the elements in each individual. For instance, communication styles will vary in a person operating from the element of fire versus earth. Fire might be loud, excitable, or harsh. On the other hand, earth might be steady, even-toned, or stubborn.

As we will see in the rest of the chapter, the elements can be formulated in pairs and opposites. It should be kept in mind that the elements are always striving for balance and harmony. Too much or too little of one or more elements is a form of imbalance. It is also important to keep in mind that balance and harmony are not static states. The universe is constantly emerging into form, being sustained and maintained for a period of time, and then eventually dissolving out of form, returning once again to the formless state. There is a quiescent restfulness between the period of form having dissolved and before form emerges. The element into and out of that all elements emerge from and return to is the element of space. As we work with the elements, the primary focus will be on balancing earth, water, air, and fire. I have included a summary in table 12.1 of the properties of the elements covered to this point with the intention that they reground the framework before we dive a little deeper.

Table 12.1 – Summary of the elements

Element	Subtle Body	Primary Lesson	Primary Principle
Earth (Prthvi)	Physical and Etheric Body (Annamaya and Pranamaya Kosha)	Grounded, embodiment in and through physical form	Stability and Solidity
Water (Ap)	Astral Body (Manomaya Kosha)	Flow, flow of emotions and Self expression	Liquidity
Air (Vayu)	Mental Body (Manomaya Kosha)	Perspective, clarity, equanimity, and increasing flexibility of consciousness	Aeriality
Fire (Agni representing fire; Rupa representing color and form)	Causal Body (Vijnanamaya Kosha)	Alignment with and expression of personal dharma (life path) through form	Form building
Space or Ether (Akasha)	Buddhic or Bliss Body (Anandamaya Kosha)	Unity, oneness, integration, balance with all the elements	Ethereality

The individual matrix

This section aims to identify your blend of the four elements from most comfortable to least comfortable. The section also begins to introduce some of the elements' characteristics that will be necessary as the practices progressively increase the challenge for restoring and maintaining balance.

Exercise 1

Of the four elements listed, circle the one that you immediately feel a strong connection and resonance with:

Earth Water Fire Air

Exercise 2

In the following list, rank numerically in order of preference (with one being the most and four being the least) where you would rather go for a weekend vacation:

- cabin in the mountains _____
- a cottage on a lakefront or beachfront _____
- rock climbing in the Sierra's _____
- visiting an active volcano _____

Exercise 3

In the following list, rank numerically from most to least (with one being the most and four being the least) which describes you best:

- hike _____
- swim _____
- hot air balloon _____
- build a fire _____

Exercise 4

Notice how you feel as you contemplate the elements. Notice sensations of discomfort, withdrawing, contracting versus expanding, opening, and relaxing. In table 12.2, rank numerically these sensations and their association with an element (with one representing sensations of the most comfort and openness and four representing sensations of the most contraction and discomfort).

Table 12.2 – Ranking of the elements

	Earth	Water	Air	Fire
Completely Comfortable				
Mostly Comfortable				
Mildly Uncomfortable				
Very Uncomfortable				

You hopefully now have a sense of which element you are most comfortable with and how you tend to think about creating your reality. This will be the foundation for working with the next stage, seeing the elements in their complementary and opposite pairs.

Combinations – Pairs and Opposites

I imagine that most readers would be familiar with the game rock-paper-scissors. The game is usually played in three rounds, with two players. After a quick countdown, each player rapidly extends their hand, neither player knowing the choice of the other, making the shape of one of the three objects. A player wins the round if their choice overcomes the other player's; for instance, a rock can overcome the scissors, or the scissors can overcome paper. The essence of the game is that it represents a set of relationships between the objects.

In a similar sense, the four elements – earth, water, air, fire – share certain relationships in which they balance or imbalance each other or are more complementary in their symbiotic relationship versus their opposite. Think of a river as an example of the complementary relationship between water and earth. A river runs along a path on the ground, between and over rocks and sand. A river does not run through the air. Conversely, if there is a forest fire, the intense heat will consume whatever water is in its path, using the water to fuel its oxygen-hungry need.

The value of understanding complementary and opposite relationships from the perspective of the elements is the insight it provides into our imbalances. It becomes possible to see more clearly areas that are blocked, why there is a lack of direction in life, and deeper insight into the dynamics of our relationships with other people, whether that be one-on-one or in various sized groups. Working with the elements is not a new concept. For instance, healing systems, such as Homeopathy and Ayurveda, have utilized these basic principles for restoring balance. In Homeopathy, the basic principle is that like and like cure, whereas, in Ayurveda, opposites reduce the imbalance and eventually lead to healing. While the application here is not specifically through herbs, similar principles for restoring balance and flow remain.

The elements are paired as follows:

1. Earth and Water are complementary
2. Air and Fire are complementary

In contrast, the elements are in opposition to each other as follows:

1. Earth is opposite to Air and Fire
2. Water is opposite to Air and Fire

3. Fire is opposite to Earth and Water
4. Air is opposite to Earth and Water

Earth and water feed each other, like the mountains that hold the rivers and streams. Water is the flow that gives life to physical reality, our creative pursuits that manifest in all the things we can see and touch with our five senses. Air and fire feed each other, like oxygen fueling the campfire. Fire is the passion and enthusiasm that gives life to the very ideas that take shape in our minds and our hearts. Too much air and not enough earth usually result in feeling ungrounded. Not enough air means it's hard to see the woods for the trees, and as a result, that is a lack of a higher perspective.

Our common use, everyday language contains expressions (aphorisms, metaphors, idioms) that, in many ways, express our innate awareness of our relationship to the elements. Looking at some of these will assist us in developing a better understanding of returning to and creating flow.

One additional consideration of the elements is that all four elements consist of a blend of the others. The primary element is the main expression and predominance of its properties. Within that are subordinate, let's say, components. These components create dimensionality and nuance to the elements, especially regarding healing and balance. If we keep in mind that the elements exist in their potential form in a state of equilibrium, any number of permutations is possible upon manifesting. This means that:

- Earth is – earth of earth, water of earth, fire of earth, air of earth
- Water is – water of water, earth of water, fire of water, air of water
- Air is – air of air, water of air, fire of air, earth of air
- Fire is – fire of fire, earth of fire, water of fire, air of fire

Although it may be simpler to say that one element is needed to balance the other, it should be kept in mind that usually, there is a primary element coupled with its secondary influence. This secondary influence can provide insight for a return to a state of balance but also be a component of the imbalance. Let's think about this in the context of emotions, for instance. Where emotions are associated primarily with the element of water, each emotion itself expresses certain qualities:

- Resentment – a slow simmering burn, like smoldering coals (fire)
- Anger – burning hotter than resentment, like a fiery eruptive volcano (water of fire)
- Exuberance – tears through a room like a tornado or a gust of wind (air of water)
- Sadness – a deep, cold, dark well (earth of water)
- Grief – small and large waves crash one on top of the other, seeming to have no end and no beginning (water of water)

As you can see, each emotion is not only about whether the water element is obstructed or flowing. The energetic formulation of each emotion offers greater depth and insight to its meaning, which in turn leads to possibilities for change.

There are countless permutations and lessons involved with working with the elements. A small sample of examples is offered below, with a symptom and remedy to illustrate one of the ways we can balance the elements. First examining the properties of the elements in table 12.3, we are directed to some of the qualities of the elements that we can then work with in the examples, in order to restore balance and harmony.

Table 12.3 – Properties of the elements

Element	Earth	Water	Air	Fire
Properties	Solid, stable, heavy, cool, warm, sluggish, slow, unmoving	Liquid, viscous, frozen, cold, hot, tepid, rapid, slow	Tasteless, odorless, colorless, thin, thick, heavy, light	Warm, hot, scorching, steaming, bright, dim, glowing, combustible
Insufficient	Stupor	Bottled up	Unclear	Unmotivated
Balanced	Grounded	Flowing	Equanimity	Transformed
Excessive	Stuck, like mud	Swamped, like under water	Suffocating, no clear view	Scorched, burned down

Too much water, not enough fire

Symptom: Stacks of paper piled everywhere; dishes piled up in the sink; piles of clothing and unfolded laundry.

Remedy: Fire is needed to burn up the excess water. With fire, excess water can be burned up, which in turn, converts the water into steam which creates motion. Fire represents motivation, the energy of which is needed to clean things up and get organized. Think about what energizes you? Perhaps playing an upbeat and energetic soundtrack or radio station while cleaning sounds like fun. If the room is dark, or it's a gloomy day, turning on some lights can help to brighten things up.

Quick tip: Think about actions or activities that inspire movement.

Too much fire, not enough water

Symptom: A fiery temper, emotions boiling over, fire burns up the water

Remedy: When fire burns, it eventually dries up any water that it comes into contact with. When emotions build up, they can generate pressure like a volcano. Suddenly, there is an eruption, with or without warning. Water needs to be allowed to flow. This calls for an appropriate channel for expressing and communicating feelings. This might involve the use of a journal to write down the feelings that have bubbled up. Talking to a trusted friend or teacher — someone who will listen without judgment, where feelings can be expressed constructively and openly. Exercise can be another powerful form of expressing feelings; the body literally pouring out through sweat emotional build up.

Quick tip: Think about actions or activities that inspire expression.

Not enough fire, too little air

Symptom: A project that at one point in time, generated excitement, and interest, now lacks direction and passion. Without enthusiasm, there is not enough momentum to keep moving forward.

Remedy: A key ingredient in making a fire is oxygen. Fire needs air to breathe. Here, fire and air support each other when brought into balance. The element of air provides the much-needed perspective to see things from a new or larger point of view. With a renewed perspective, it's possible to see what direction to take, whether it means staying the course or changing tack, breathing renewed vigor into the project. With direction refocused, and wind beneath one's wings, the fire of motivation is renewed once again. Perspective and insight are often sought in contemplative practice such as meditation. Finding clarity often results when the mind is held in a state a calm equanimity. It is possible to generate insight through dialogue that seeks active reflection and guidance. An individual such as a mentor, coach, or advisor can provide another point of view.

Quick tip: Thing about actions that free up space.

Too much earth, not enough water and fire

Symptom: A large project looms ahead. There are feelings of being overwhelmed, swamped, and eventually, buried under its weight.

Remedy: If we think about dirt that has been flooded it generally turns to mud. Dirt, and indeed mud, is heavy enough on its own. With excess water further weight is added. In this scenario, all that excess water needs to be dried out. We know that heating water with fire turns it into steam, and eventually, the water will evaporate. We also know that the energy of fire provides light and fuel. We have multiple elements that need to be balanced. Air offers clarity and perspective for seeing what the steps are, and which ones to take next. A journal exercise is one type of practice that can support the need to get clear. Slowing down when feeling overwhelmed is another step, and this may involve taking a long walk to settle the mind and the body. Movement practices that integrate mindfulness such as Tai Chi or gentle Hatha Yoga, can also support moving from feeling overwhelmed to calm inner stillness. With more space and life force available, it's once again possible to regenerate feelings of motivation and enthusiasm.

Quick tip: Think about activities or actions that inspire solidity, movement, and illumination.

Relationships

Another area to consider of the elements' role is within the context of relationships. For simplicity, I will refer to the interaction as occurring between two individuals rather than the more complex situations of groups. In the context of two people, the principles remain the same for groups. Between two individuals, a relationship can be thought of as a container. The container holds together all the non-material information of the dynamic between these two individuals. For as long as the relationship exists, the container holds the exchanges of energy between these two individuals. In itself, the container holds a template of the learning and growth that has been undertaken jointly. The elements, when they exist in their non-material form, are energy. So too is the soul an energy. Therefore, we can talk about the nature of a relationship from the perspective of the interaction of the elements as part of the container itself. Blockages, feeling stuck, patterns that repeat without resolution, communication styles; can all be viewed from the perspective of the elements.

A person who is quick to temper may generally have fire as a predominant element. Therefore, in situations of stress or when an unresolved inner pattern is triggered, their default could be to respond from fire. Conversely, the other person who possibly is more sensitive responds in the same way water would if approached with fire. Water retreats when a fire is near. There is a fear of being burned up or scorched.

No matter the dynamics of the elements, in general, one of the lessons of any relationship is learning to develop more compassion for each other. The value of skillful embodiment of compassion is that it takes us out of the habit-driven tendencies and conditioning of the mind and personality and instead elevates us to our higher potentials for seeing each other as our true Selves. At this level, it's possible to see one another in our true form, as the essence and energy of the Source. As with our own development of the subtle bodies, so too are our relationships invited to grow to their highest potential. A relationship that has found a union and balance of a higher order recognizes "no barrier, no difference" and "no separation" (Besant. p. 182). The experience of oneness is a bliss experience, and how beautiful is that in the sacredness of a deep relationship!

Summary
It is no small endeavor to reach the state of union that is a "bliss experience," to live from it and embody it. The natural human

tendency is for individuals to project some inner thought or feeling about some prior experience, or about someone else, onto another person. These projections are stories that separate us from realizing a higher perspective and embodying a greater state of union, which in essence, is an unrecognized inner drive at the core of every human being. In pulling back the curtain of the stories we tell ourselves, it becomes increasingly more and more realizable that union and harmony are not only within our grasp, but an embodied lived experience.

Practice – Inner inquiry

What happens when we find ourselves not in a state of balance, or we don't feel quite centered, unsure what the next step is, or even what we need? A simple practice of asking "what is needed of me?" could be just the remedy. In general, the answers we seek are within ourselves – our hearts and minds. The practice is essentially a reminder and a call back to the wisdom each of us has within ourselves. This is not to say we should not seek outside of ourselves. Rather, we re-familiarize ourselves by engaging with our own inner compass. Looking at it from the perspective of the elements, if what is needed is the enthusiasm and passion of the fire element, we can look within to ask what step we could take in pursuit of igniting that flame. The answer may surprise us when coming from the light and wisdom of the soul rather than the part of the mind that tries to come up with a picture that is often unsatisfactory. In any moment when there is uncertainty, worry, doubt, or just plain old feelings of being stuck, the practice invites us to slow down and pause. Just as there exists a natural liminal space between each inhale and exhale, there is a liminal space between this moment and the next. As we slow down and pause, becoming quiet and still, we can feel our way into that dynamic space of possibility. Here, in this dynamic stillness, we find a space in which time seems almost to stand still. As the mind becomes quiet, we ask a single question: *what is needed of me in this moment?* And then we watch, gradually, as rays of possibilities open up within our inner visual field. As we watch, one ray may light up more than the others. Or, there may be some other indicator that pursuing one possibility over another is most in flow. It could be a sound, a smell of sweet perfume, or celebration fireworks. The important thing is to watch as the soul speaks and then follow.

Practice – Welcoming the elements

As we have now learned, each element has its own unique properties that distinguish it from the others, including some portion of the other elements within itself. As we begin to incorporate a worldview from the perspective of the five elements, welcoming them into our hearts and minds creates connection and invites the possibility of collaboration with them. Even though a hurricane may take down a hundred trees, earth knows that exposure to the light of the sun will give new energy for seeds of new trees to grow, the space necessary for that growth to happen. The elements work together in a constant state of creating, maintaining, and returning to balance. As we welcome the elements, we invite their wisdom and teaching to illuminate our hearts and minds, that we may each live in greater harmony and unity. As a simple practice, we work with each element individually, seeing them in our inner mind's eye represented as a color. In a similar way that we might imagine the energetic center of a particular *chakra*, we envision an element as a single, round point. This point is like a *bindu*, a special focal point that concentrates and stills the mind. Focusing on the *bindu*, we use a color to denote which particular element we are focusing upon, its energy, and qualities, with an intention to welcome and embody these qualities. We use green for earth, blue for water, yellow for air, red for fire, and translucent white for space. Over time, the elements may offer themselves to you in a form and color that better symbolizes your relationship to them. In the meantime, we invite you to use this color library from our own practice as a starting point.

The colors may remain the same, but they may also change. Focus on one element at a time, one practice session at a time. For example, you might sit for five minutes or twenty. It largely depends on the meditator's experience. Beginning meditators can start with smaller increments, slowly building the mental flexibility of concentrated focus necessary for longer meditation sessions. Focusing on the element's qualities and properties opens the mind to become completely immersed and absorbed therein. Generally, a good practice is to keep a journal, noting what was experienced and observed without becoming attached from one session to the next. The journal helps to record and then let go. It's important that we have no expectation of repeating a prior experience in any meditation session. Any expectation itself becomes an obstacle. Beginners' mind is always a sound practice.

Practice – Element balancing

There are two basic principles to remember when an element needs to be balanced. The first principle brings in the energy of the opposite element. The second principle brings in more of the same element's energy. A desk buried under mounds of paperwork and spread out so much that they threaten to spill over the edge symbolizes the water element needing to be restrained, possibly by the element of fire. By bringing in organizational tools that create order and stability, as well as excitement to create a renewed space, the opposite energies of earth and fire both absorb and burn up all the excess water. Creating organizational order does not mean that one should rush out to purchase all new office tools. That would be another form of imbalance, such as in the case of burning a hole in one's pocket (excess fire). In essence, two simple questions can be asked:

1. Which element is out of balance?
2. Which element(s) do I need to draw upon to restore balance?

It's important to watch, wait, see what shows up, and stay open to receiving inner guidance without rushing to assumptions or judgments. Notice when the answers initiate a feeling of openness in the heart, mind, and body and are accompanied by an influx of more energy, vitality, and expansion. As a general rule of thumb, whatever guidance is received, let it sit for a day or two, and then check back in to see if anything has changed or stayed the same.

Practice – Developing heart consciousness

The lotus flower has long been an important symbol, particularly in Buddhism. It represents our capacity to rise above the human physical realm of attachment and desire to the realm of an enlightened and awakened mind. In this meditation practice, the energetic heart center is visualized as a white lotus flower. The color white has often been a symbol portraying purity and enlightenment. Thus, the lotus flower combined with the color of white, we imagine drawing into ourselves the qualities of open-mindedness and compassion. In the light spectrum, the color white is formed as a combination of all colors. We can thus think of an additional symbol represented by this white lotus flower, namely the path of union. When we open ourselves up to the path of union, to see the fundamental connection of all life as one that is shared interdependently, we naturally open our capacity to be compassionate and loving. This is a formative step in developing the skills and the energetic heart muscle of compassion.

To begin this meditation, find a relatively quiet place free of distraction. Settle the body into a comfortable and easy meditation posture, slowing down the breath, gradually relaxing the body's muscles. Gathering focus, attention, and energy invite the thinking mind to drop into stillness, watching as thoughts fall from awareness like pebbles settling into the soft floor of the ocean. Gradually draw in the light of the awakened mind, watching as awareness becomes clearer and calmer. Bring the awakened mind into the heart center as you visualize a white lotus flower. Merge your consciousness with this lotus flower, as if seeing yourself not only in the lotus but becoming the lotus itself. Hold this state of focus for a few minutes to start. With more experience, this can be extended to a half-hour. Whatever the duration, do not try to force anything. The practice is all about opening and expanding. Anything that is forced or strained will have the opposite effect, which is to contract. After completing this portion of the practice, you are ready to return to ordinary waking consciousness. Let go of the image of the lotus flower. Return your attention to your body and your breath, becoming aware of the inhale and exhale. Take a few more breaths as you gradually start to move the body around, such as standing up to stretch the legs or arms. Slowly, open your eyes, taking in your surroundings. Gradually return to the routine of your day or evening.

Chapter 12

Heart Consciousness

Psychology and ethic are not the same. The science of psychology is the result of the study of the mind. The science of ethic is the result of the study of conduct, so as to bring about the harmonious relation of one to another. Ethic is a science of life, and not an investigation into the nature of mind and the methods by which the powers of the mind may be developed and evolved.

(Annie Besant, *An Introduction to Yoga*)

Heart consciousness is a collection of attitudes and values that, when put into daily practice, contribute toward a life that is lived in service for the greater good, which in turn contributes to a greater universal harmony. Part of human nature is the inborn instinct to have concern and care for the well-being of others. Heart consciousness amplifies this in practical steps. In turn, the circle for whom we care is widened, opening to larger and larger groups of human and sentient beings. Harmony recognizes the universal principle of the interdependence of all beings and phenomena from which heart consciousness is born.

In some traditions, the energetic heart is thought of as the true seat of wisdom. It is typically associated with attitudes and qualities such as unconditional love, kindness, generosity, compassion, empathy, fellowship, kinship, and tenderness. These attitudes are essentially an antidote to the false self that believes it is separate from everyone and everything.

Selfishness is born from the notion of a separate self. There is a distinction to be made between the self-care of only oneself versus the self-care that considers the greater good of all – the *all* of which includes oneself as well. There is an ideal balance to be found wherein an individual can balance the integrity of their needs and self-hood while simultaneously considering the needs of others. Selfishness closes the circle of connection and harmony, whereas, as it gradually dissolves, so too are the boundaries of separation.

Out of harmony arises joy, a natural expression of participation with the flow and balance of the Universe. Harmony, therefore, is an ideal that everyone is invited to align themselves with or not. As we come closer to this ideal, joy and fulfillment increase. The further away from the ideal we move, the more that dissatisfaction and suffering increase.

In the Yoga Sūtras of Patanjali, a benefit to cultivating attitudes aligned with the ideal of harmony is suggested. Sutra 1.33: "The mind becomes clarified by cultivating attitudes of friendliness, compassion, gladness and indifference respectively towards happiness, misery, virtue and vice" (Taimni, I.K. p. 85). In other words, cultivating these attitudes acts as an antidote to mental illusions that obscure the nature of the true Self, obstacles that stand in the way of experiencing the genuine joy and fulfillment of the true Self.

The way toward harmony encompasses two processes that work in tandem together. One system involves living from the set of heart-based values regularly. The other consists of adopting a set of values that inform embodied living from the ideal of harmony.

Values are more of the action-oriented components of a belief or set of beliefs. As stated earlier in the book, thoughts create reality, and beliefs are very much a part of what we think.

As we examine the values laid out below, I wish to distinguish between the existence of personal values and universal values. The reason this distinction is important has to do with acknowledging how people choose to live their life differently from others. Universal values should not contradict these choices but instead respect the free will of every individual. I hope it will be evident that this is not in contradiction to being aligned with the ideal of harmony.

Universal values

Five universal values are outlined herein, and while there may be more, these feel to us to be the most impactful and in no way impinge on the will and choice of an individual's personal values. These are tolerance, non-violence, compassion, empathic joy, and forgiveness.

Tolerance

I define tolerance as *the magnanimous generosity of an open heart and mind, that, without prejudice, patiently welcomes and accepts that from which it differs.* The human tendency is to withdraw or turn away when faced with something that brings up sensations of discomfort. What if we instead accepted the challenge, leaning into the discomfort with patience and an open mind? What if, instead, we look at the moment as an invitation to expand our capacity to be a little more open-hearted? What if we apply these questions to our interactions with people we don't know?

A core principle of tolerance is acceptance. As a value, tolerance accepts that my beliefs, my views, and my outlook on life are different from someone else's. In accepting this difference, I do not try to change the other person's views by force or by the pressure of my own personal will to influence them. Tolerance invites me to consider these differences, even if our personal values are not in alignment with each other. Tolerance builds a bridge and is the first step in welcoming these differences into a space where it might be possible to discover who someone is. It becomes an invitation to walk toward rather than away from one another.

Adopting the value of tolerance is greatly supported in developing or expanding a number of other core skills. These include active listening, listening with non-judgment, empathy, compassion, and generosity. These skills are addressed throughout the rest of this chapter.

Non harming

A core value in Indian philosophy is called *ahimsā*, often translated as non-violence or non-harming. However, it is not exclusive to this system of beliefs. Rather, as a universal value, it can also be found within many of the world's spiritual traditions such as Buddhism, Judaism, Christianity, and Islam. At its root, non-harmfulness or non-violence extends beyond simply *do not kill* or *do not take the life of another being*. It also means "not willfully inflicting any injury, suffering or pain on any living creature, by word, thought, or action" and simultaneously recognizing the "underlying unity of life" (Taimni, I.K. p. 209–210). Adding to Taimni's definition, it could also be said that suffering or pain inflicted can vary in intensity, depending upon the force with which it is motivated. It is also true to say that a thought, word, or action can unintentionally cause some form of harm, even though there was no motivation to do so. The last point contains an important key in cultivating a value and attitude of non-harming, namely, motivation.

What if we adopted the value of non-harming? How would this shift our thoughts and attitudes on a daily basis? What consequences would this have for ourselves and others? A simple but profound teaching ascribed to Mahatma Gandhi says that one needs to *begin with oneself to see a change in the world*. I would argue that the change which begins with each individual is whether we are motivated toward an ideal of harmony and unity or not.

If we are indeed motivated toward harmony and unity, two things are important to consider if non-harming is to be embodied daily. The first involves mindful awareness of one's thoughts, emotions, and words, from which action naturally follows. The second recognizes the unity of all life when we stop to consider the consequences of our actions and their impact on oneself, others, and Nature. How do we translate this into actions whereby our thoughts, beliefs, feelings, and needs are communicated, which adds to a greater harmony and unity for all?

Language, both written and spoken word, continues to be one of the most important tools used by humans to convey thoughts and ideas. And it is also one of the tools most easily misused. A simple task such as asking where to find the nearest restroom takes on a new meaning when asking the same question in a language different from one's own. The challenges of conveying and exchanging thoughts, feelings, and needs are amplified the more complex the ideas are. Add to this the unique make-up of each individual's experiences and communication skills; it's no wonder that communication can be a veritable minefield. Despite the challenges, it is possible to navigate the terrain of communication in ways that increase harmony, peace, and unity.

We find practical and common-sense guidance from Annie Besant when she writes, "Let him speak the truth, let him speak the pleasing, let him not speak an unpleasing truth, nor speak a pleasing falsehood; this is the ancient law" (Besant, A. p. 234). What would it look like if we turned Annie Besant's statements above into questions? I have found this to be a useful practice over the years, of turning a phrase or statement into a question, which leads me to discovering more insight and fresh perspectives. In this practice, introduced to me some years ago by Kurt Leland [2011–2022], in any given moment, we ask ourselves three questions:

1. Is it useful?
2. Is it kind?
3. Is it true?

It's no coincidence that we have the axiom as part of common language; *think before you speak!* Whether inwardly as in one's inner voice or outwardly, what we say has power. Inner dialogue is how we speak to ourselves. Outer dialogue is how we speak to others either about ourselves, about them, or about others. In whichever direction words are targeted, the energy behind them has real impact and consequence. In 1999, Dr. Masaru Emoto's book, *The Messages of Water*, presented a series of photographs he had taken of frozen water crystals, each one expressing the unique ways in which water expresses itself. His experiments developed further, examining the effect that various kinds of music, as well as certain words, had on the formation of water crystals. His experiments were remarkable. Under a microscope, beautifully shaped crystals could be seen in water that had been exposed to positive phrases such as *thank you*. By contrast, however, water exposed to negative phrases such as *you fool* showed deformed and misshapen crystals (Emoto, M. p. 45). With these experiments, the unseen was made visible – words, whether in the form of an unspoken thought or orally expressed, have the power to affect not only ourselves but also the field of energy around us. Therefore, in practice, breaking down each of the above three questions, it's possible to examine their application in all dimensions of daily living.

As I understand it, *usefulness* can be examined by looking at *dharma* and *motivation*. In the first instance, we ask ourselves: do my thoughts, words, or actions help guide the other person closer to, or further away from, their *dharma*, which is their path? In the second instance, we examine our *motivation* behind our thoughts, words, and actions, asking ourselves: are they altruistic and for the greater good, or are they self-serving? Let's review these questions from the perspective of Dr. Emoto's experiments. The experiments are useful in that they demonstrate how thoughts and words physically affect the targeted subject. Consider how telling someone that they are smart and capable supports them in discovering their dharma, whereas in contrast telling someone that they are unintelligent, and incapable does the opposite. Usefully, we can apply these same questions to ourselves as they relate to inner dialogue.

We find three key attributes within kindness: considerate, friendly, and supportive. This brings to mind the film *Pay it Forward* (2000), a story of a boy who started a movement of goodwill. The film depicted how goodwill and kindness, motivated by altruism, could greatly benefit both the giver and the receiver. It also demonstrated the impact these actions had on the wider community. One of the most poignant elements the movie highlighted is that kindness is an infinite resource, available to everyone, and can be drawn upon anytime. It also demonstrated that kindness does not require that a person reaches into their wallet. Smiling at someone, even if you are strangers to one another, can be just the salve they need at that moment to realize that someone else sees them.

In practice, we are always circulating between kindness to oneself, kindness to others, and kindness to the environment. I remember when I was quite young, maybe a little older than five or six years old when I was outside in my grandparents' garden. I had picked a few leaves off a large shrub, which instantly oozed a milky white substance. In his firm but gentle voice, my grandfather came over to me and told me that the milky substance was the plant crying; that by pulling its leaves, I was causing it pain. Plants, when wounded or injured, will move to protect themselves and heal the affected area to prevent disease or further damage. Human beings are not much different; cleaning a wound on the skin and applying a Band-Aid to support the body's healing mechanism. It was an important lesson that taught me at a young age the value of care and consideration for the environment and how my actions have consequences. My grandfather's lesson highlights the fourth attribute of kindness: patience. My grandfather had recognized that I had yet to understand the consequences of my actions fully. He provided me with a different perspective with simple, clear, and calm language. It was then up to me to step into a greater understanding and relationship with the plants.

Equally important is the practice of inner kindness, how we relate to ourselves. One way to monitor this is a mindfulness practice of observing our internal dialogue. When writing this book (2020–2021), an inspired Pixar film called *Soul* (2020) was released. One of the main characters is a soul named 22, and as we watch the story around their character unfold, we come to observe their inner dialogue. We eventually learn that long-held thoughts and beliefs, reiterated in their internal dialogue, have held them back from taking an important next step in their journey. Once the character realized that none of those thoughts and beliefs were true, it became possible to replace them with words and thoughts rooted in kindness. As life force increased, it became possible for them to take their next step. And that step opened into a joy of new possibilities.

The third pillar of communication is truth. Naturally, we might think of the opposite to truth: dishonesty or lying. However, truth encompasses much more than honesty, so I became curious about how a dictionary might define it. Instead of a clear definition, I found that truth was described in terms of its inherent qualities, namely, "the quality or state of being true" ("Truth," n.d.). What, then, is a universal truth? For something to be universal, it means "including or covering all or a whole collectively or distributively without limit or exception" ("Universal," n.d). We can, therefore, say that a universal truth is collectively true for an entire collective, such as all of society. For example, an accepted universal truth is that the earth revolves around the sun; the sun rises in the cardinal east and sets in the cardinal west. These truths do not change based on circumstances or location; these examples apply whether or not you live in the Southern or Northern Hemisphere of the planet.

Truth is not absolute. Not being absolute is an important distinction, especially when motivated to communicate or relate from a value of non-harmfulness. In other words, my truth is not your truth. Truth is another way of saying *dharma* – *my dharma is not your dharma, and your dharma is not mine.* One of the ways I have come to think about truth is simply as a wise guide. The wise guide directs a path toward an authentic alignment with my soul and the universe. The universe includes whoever or whatever I am in contact with at any given moment. The path is the particular set of lessons that each individual learns as part of the return journey back to the Source. More often than not, conflict arises when one individual attempts, knowingly or unknowingly, to assert their truth *over* that of the other person. A common situation between a parent and a child involves the parent's insistence that the child follows a particular profession. This insistence often disregards the child's own inner promptings or desires until years later, when the child realizes that they are not fulfilled and makes a change. On a smaller scale, it can be all too easy to fall into the trap of giving advice, especially unsolicited, from the perspective of what would be true and right for the advice-giver, but not for the person to whom the advice is being given.

Moment to moment, we have access to the soul's wisdom illuminating the path. Opening up to the moment in kindness, and drawing in the soul's wisdom, leads to harmony. And harmony leads to joy. If we are to cultivate non-harming, we can use the three questions posed above – true, kind, useful, in daily practice with ourselves and others.

Compassion

Compassion and pity seek, as does all love to lessen the distance between itself and its object, to raise its object towards itself.
(Besant, A. p. 244)

Annie Besant gives us good direction for how we might begin to think about, cultivate and practice compassion. Let's start with an intention, as suggested in Besant's words: to reduce the distance between myself and anything that appears as outside myself. The first thing this intention implies is dissolving a perceived boundary of separation. It is so often forgotten that more connects and joins us than divides or separates us. Compassion loosens these boundaries. An essential ingredient of compassion is understanding. It could be said that there are four components to understanding: comprehension, consideration, perception, and realization. These are building blocks necessary for an important attitude and skill called empathy.

An early notion of empathy finds its roots in the German term *einfühlung*. Briefly, einfühlung is the *willingness* and the *capacity* of a person to *feel into or project* themselves into the experience of another *person, object, place, or other sentient beings* (Ganczarek, et al., 2018, 141).

This description can be broken down into three questions, each one a cognizable step:

1. Am I willing to try to understand the other person's point of view or experience?
2. Am I willing to be vulnerable?
3. Am I willing to feel into the experience, using not only the faculty of mind but inner sense perceptions?

With the first question, we open ourselves to the recognition that the other person has a worldview and life story that is different from ours and brought them to this moment in which you are meeting. This is true whether the person is in front of you or reading about a character in a book. It does not mean that you should or even could know the person's entire history. The step is about stepping outside of one's usual point of view. It uses imagination as if you could teleport yourself into a different time, space, and experience.

With the second question, we consider our willingness to be open. But we do this through the lens of skill-level, which means the ability to stay grounded and centered within oneself. When we are grounded and centered in ourselves, it is usually easier to open up to and remain open to others. The more skilled we are at staying centered, the easier it is to open the space for compassion, including oneself.

The third question invites us to feel into the experience or situation of the other, which grants us the lens of their point of view. Instead of relying solely on the mind's capacity to problem-solve as a way to generate insight and understanding, which is a typical Western viewpoint, an Eastern approach suggests using felt senses such as intuition, regarding them as valid tools for learning. This approach means emptying your cup as a vehicle for opening up to a greater realm of possibilities.

Felt senses can be thought of as five ways of knowing reality (*pancha jnanendriya*). In someone else's case, it is the reality they themselves are experiencing. These senses are connected to the five organs of action (*pancha karmmendriya*), both of which are connected to the five elements as they appear in their subtle (*tanmatras*) and material forms (*pancha mahabhutas*).

Felt senses tap into our abilities:

- to listen inwardly (ear, sound)
- to connect beyond physical touch (skin, touch)
- to see inwardly beyond what is visible to the naked eye (sight, vision)
- to get a sense of the flavor of the experience (taste, variety)
- to digest it all, taking in everything the way the breath comes in and goes out (smell, nose)

These felt senses are in and available to each of us. They are developed in similar ways as you might build muscles in the body – with exercise. We identify three skills that cultivate an open heart and compassion and develop the felt senses:

1. Mental equipoise
2. Active listening
3. Selfless service

Mental equipoise is a state of mind in which a person is able to remain present, alert, and neutral without becoming detached, aloof, or cold. Equanimity or evenness of mind develops through concentration and single-pointed focus. The basis of this can be found in basic mind training. With a continuous steady flow of concentration and non-judgmental awareness, an individual is able to remain in the present moment as both the witness and the participant of their own inner experience. I would argue that this is foundational if we are to cultivate a capacity not only to hold multiple perspectives but to do so with a neutral mind. At any given point, all that is being asked of us is to be present and open, like the wide blue sky.

Active listening is an agile practice where a person refrains from projecting their expectations, feelings, or thoughts onto the other person when in active listener mode. There are natural human tendencies to want to interrupt or interject with the intention, consciously or not, to make the conversation or situation about oneself. As His Holiness the Dalai Lama has said:

> We do not stop to consider the complexity of a given situation. Our tendency is to rush in and do what seems to promise the shortest route to satisfaction. But in doing so, all too frequently we deprive ourselves of the opportunity for a greater degree of fulfillment. When we act to fulfill our immediate desires without taking into account others' interests, we undermine the possibility of lasting happiness.

(His Holiness the Dalai Lama, p. 52–53)

Active listening invites each person to be present in the moment with no agenda or expectations, to show up to the best of their ability, without thinking about anything else. It's natural for the mind to drift. That's why meditation that teaches single-pointed concentration is so beneficial. It helps develop this necessary capacity to stay in the moment without becoming distracted. If one can remain present and undistracted, the greater the possibility exists to track what is being said, both the verbal and the non-verbal language. You are able to remain attentive when a pause is needed, either for one or both of you to absorb or to create a break so that reflection and clarification can take place. A mindful pause, in turn, deepens the experience. It's in this space in which it's possible for a person to be fully seen and fully heard, which is a universal human need. Non-violent communication is a practice that Marshall B. Rosenberg developed. His work is an excellent resource for developing these skills and well worth reading his writing on the subject.

Selfless service is the act of considering the needs of others, not above yours but in conjunction with yours. Needs, in general, are universal. Every individual and every sentient being has a set of needs. As needs arise and are fulfilled, there is a feeling of increasing satisfaction. In small ways and large, we can become more self-aware – aware of our actions' impact on others. We can choose to be less self-centered and selfish and instead selfless, loving, and thoughtful. Being service-oriented can take many forms. It can be a small act, like offering someone with fewer groceries than you to take your place as next in line.

There are, however, a few things that can get in the way of becoming more service-oriented:

1. A belief such as *I was here first*.
2. A belief in scarcity is a fear of not enough whether that is time, money, resources, support, etc.
3. A belief of entitlement such as *I deserve this more than someone else.*

If we drop these beliefs, we return to Annie Besant's words on compassion and love, reducing the distance between self and other. As we ascend our own ladder of spiritual development, and in the process developing compassion for others, "we must learn how to embrace and understand the suffering of others, one person at a time, to see ourselves reflected in others, as if each suffering being were a stage of our own development that we might have left behind" (Leland, K. p. 191).

Empathetic Joy

Some cultures, more than others, emphasize a value of competition and survival of the fittest. This idea has an unfortunate consequence of engendering competition, fueled by the beliefs of getting ahead at any cost and that the ends justify the means. The opposite of competition is an attitude that values and celebrates collaboration. Collaboration is the willingness to give and receive help where needed. Empathetic joy is completely opposite to competition. It is the capacity and willingness to feel into the joy that someone else is experiencing as they fulfill their dharma and any area in their life aligned with the core of their Being.

Competitiveness, with perfectionism as the other side of the coin, can be a difficult blindspot to see. It is especially true if one's values are inconsistent with this attitude. If, for instance, one values humbleness and teamwork, it may not be easy to acknowledge that you secretly want to win that next bowling game.

To truly celebrate the joy someone else is experiencing means feeling unselfish and genuinely pleased for them. You rejoice with them when they get a strike (in bowling – knocking down all the pins on the first roll of the bowling ball). There is a sincere and genuine desire to celebrate another person's growth, even participating where you can in supporting to lift them up to that next higher level. Competition does the opposite of this.

Whenever we compare ourselves to someone else, it takes away something from both of us. It takes away the joy and celebration of their achievement and the opportunity it could have created for becoming closer. And it takes away from yourself in all the ways that you don't think you're good enough or think you have to be somehow better than they are to achieve as much or more.

The antidote to all this is admiration. It means to be in wonder and awe of the other person, allowing all that light and beauty that's radiating to flow through you. Celebrate your own achievements without the need or desire for approval or recognition.

Forgiveness

The value of forgiveness resides in how it frees up tangled energies that have kept people stuck in the past and unable to move forward in the moment and into the future. Forgiveness is composed of several values and attitudes, two of which we have already covered, namely understanding and tolerance. To understand the value of forgiveness, however, I believe it's important to examine why forgiveness is needed and, therefore, how it serves as a universal value.

To forgive something that is or was perceived as some wrongdoing would have preceded it. In general, blaming someone or something, including oneself, for this perceived wrongdoing, essentially sets off the chain of events, the entanglement of energies that forgiveness removes. It is important to keep in mind that forgiveness does not mean that certain behaviors like murder are condoned. However, it provides a vehicle in which reconciliation is possible and a way forward that enables the parties involved to learn and grow. Forgiveness, therefore, keeps the learning process going rather than remaining stuck.

Blame places something like a bind on oneself and or the other person. We can blame ourselves for something we did or said, feeling guilty or ashamed, and then ruminate how we are somehow not good enough or not lovable. My husband and I often use a term to free oneself in this situation: *forgive your lesser knowing self.* This statement means you permit yourself to reconcile this past experience in order to free yourself of the limitations that the bind of blame places upon you. It becomes possible for insight and understanding to develop in the process, a necessary step (or series of steps) before the process completes itself. In the final moment, a sense of calm acceptance arises to let you know that the lesson is now complete.

This process is a little more complex when it involves one or more people other than yourself. In general, though, the mechanism is the same. In group dynamics involving two or more people, responsibility is the lesson of what each person involved contributes to the situation or event. It's a contribution that could, in some ways, be compared to something like a potluck. You don't know what everyone else is bringing to eat, just as they don't know what you're bringing. And, each of you may have some opinions about those contributions, favorable or otherwise.

The universal value of forgiveness allows every individual to realize and remember that we are all in a system of learning and growth. Expanding on the notion that an eye for an eye turns the whole world blind, Besant's words and perspective offer us sage counsel:

Vindictiveness and revengefulness are the opposites of the readiness to forgive, which we have seen is a part of magnanimity, and they perpetuate troubles, keeping them alive when they might die by forgetfulness. The wish to return an injury suffered by inflicting an injury in return is a sign of complete ignorance of the working of the law. A man who suffers an injury should think that he has inflicted an injury on another in the past, and that his own fault comes back to him in the injury now inflicted upon himself. Thus he closes the account. But if he revenges himself now, he will in the future again suffer the equivalent of the revenge he takes on his enemy. For, that enemy will not be likely to think that he has been justly punished and will nurse revenge again, and so the chain of claim and counter-claim will continue endlessly. The only way to get rid of an enemy is to forgive him; revengefulness stores up trouble for the future, which will inevitably come to the revengeful person; and the injuries we suffer now are only our own revenge coming home to ourselves. No one can wound us unless our own past places a weapon in his hands. Let a student remember this when someone injuries him; let him pay his debt like an honest man and be done with it.

(Besant, A. p. 240)

In other words, cultivating the value of forgiveness has positive, life force enhancing benefits. These benefits include oneself, others, and the entire community. Forgiveness has a positive impact on a person's overall health and well-being which, according to Dr. Fred Luskin and his fellow researchers "can reduce stress, blood pressure, anger, depression, and hurt, and it can increase optimism, hope, compassion, and physical vitality" (Luskin, 2004). In other words, learning to forgive is an essential component of a healthy relationship eco-system, inwardly and outwardly, and "is good for both your mental and physical well-being and your relationships" (Luskin, Dr. F. p. xv). On a national and international scale, we can find examples of the importance of forgiveness and its possibilities in the restorative justice process, such as The Truth and Reconciliation Commission. Established in South Africa at the end of Apartheid, it was seen as a vital step in bringing healing to the people directly affected and the country as a whole. Forgiveness, in essence, is an essential part of healing. The act of forgiveness restores us to an experience of wholeness, and ultimately, unity.

Mental attitudes

Adopting certain mental attitudes brings us into closer alignment with the above-mentioned universal values. We can follow this useful advice given by the Dalai Lama: "If a room is too hot, the only way to reduce the heat is to introduce cold. Just as heat and cold oppose each other, so, too, do mental states such as anger and compassion. To the extent you develop one, the other decreases. This is the way that counterproductive states of mind are reduced, and finally removed" (His Holiness the Dalai Lama. p. 9). Although many other attitudes have been identified throughout the book that speak to this advice, the two attitudes specifically identified here for reflection are, grace and gratitude.

Grace

Grace flows throughout the universe and is a gentle force that embraces all beings. Recognizing the presence of this energy is a mental attitude that opens up to a higher state of consciousness. Behind the energy of grace is recognizing the existence of a higher power supporting and guiding everyone and everything. It places you back in touch with the interconnectedness and oneness of all life.

Closing your eyes, you might imagine this like the rays of the sun just before dusk. The sunset light casts a soft, golden glow, not too hot but just enough to warm the skin tenderly. As you imagine this light, you might open up to it more and more to feel it fill you up, lifting you gently into the warm embrace of grace.

Gratitude

Gratitude moves us from what we think we don't have toward what we do have. Instead of what may be lacking or insufficient, there's abundance. It puts us back in touch with all the beauty within us and around us. Gratitude is an invitation to be thankful for where you are in the moment, what you have, the people in your life, and so forth. A simple practice, to begin with, might be to end the day reflecting upon all the things for which you are grateful. It might be the smile you received from the shop assistant or the driver who waited so you could cross a busy intersection. Gradually, the more we reflect upon that for which we are grateful, the natural result is how it opens the door of the heart. With an open heart, it's possible to be more receptive to the love and help that is always available, and in return, to share this with others.

Summary

Outer harmony begins with inner harmony. The challenge we all face is aligning ourselves with our core values and living from them. Thoughts, words, and actions gradually need to be brought into alignment, which is a life lesson for each person. All we can ever do is take one step, one moment at a time. Each step is an invitation to step in a larger and truer sense of oneself.

Closing Thoughts

In January 2020, a quickly developing global pandemic was unfolding thousands of miles across the ocean, far from home. It quickly became a seismic world event that touched every living being on the planet. For many people, the pandemic interrupted how day-to-day life was being lived. I saw this as the force of Shiva rippling out, breaking down very old, ingrained patterns, many of which for a long time have had severely negative impacts in hundreds of areas of life. Climate change was among the many at the top of my list. If there were ever a time when the human collective was experiencing something akin to time slowing down or even stopping, the pandemic that began in 2020 was such a vehicle.

This book was born out of this time, a time in which humanity was confronted with big questions of how to unite at a time of great universal need collectively. Scientists worldwide quickly set to work, racing to develop a vaccine. In recorded human history, the vaccines created were the quickest it has ever been, a testament to the kind of unity possible when human beings realize the power of working together instead of against one another. The pandemic also unveiled in stark view many atrocities that could no longer be ignored: poverty, institutionalized racism, marginalization of minorities, climate change, the illusion of competition, income inequality, abuse of power, and more.

Systems and ways of thinking that have long been in place were brought into question. An opportunity to learn, grow and change in the direction of more care, concern, and greater unity in part is what the pandemic put on offer. As we know it, reality is individual and collective and not mutually exclusive. My actions, your actions, our actions affect one another. We are universally interdependent – a fundamental truth. To be human, at its simplest, is to learn and grow. Within the framework of learning and growth, there are choices, the primary of which is to ask at least this one question: "how do my individual thoughts and actions contribute to a greater or lesser harmony?" Only each individual can answer this question for themselves.

We can embrace the lessons we are given or resist them. The degree to which we embrace each step along our path determines the level of satisfaction and joy we experience. The more we understand and know ourselves, the more awake we are to our core true Self, the greater the flow of life force. With every increase in the flow of life force, we come closer to experiencing ever-increasing fulfillment and satisfaction. This is a collective benefit – when one person suffers, the world feels that suffering; when one person experiences joy, the world feels that joy.

The more that each of us wakes up to the realization that we are so much more than the brain's chemical processes and an imperfect body, the greater the possibility for the collective consciousness to rise to its fullest potential. We can only do this one step at a time, and in the process, hopefully leaving as light a touch on the Earth as possible. My hope is that this small volume contributes in some way to the elevation of consciousness, that we may all live in ideal harmony and joy with ourselves and with all sentient beings.

About the Author

Nicole Goott immigrated in 2004 from Johannesburg, South Africa, at the age of twenty-four to pursue a growing inner call to not only discover but ultimately, follow her dharma. Unsatisfied with working in the financial services sector, Nicole embraced the voice of her true Self and the life of a mystic, teacher and healer. For more than a decade, Nicole has passionately taught yoga, meditation and a spiritual practice of self-discovery in group classes, workshops and intensives both publicly and privately. Nicole lives with her husband in the tranquil woods of New Hampshire, exploring the vast range of hiking trails, especially when the weather is mild and there are no mosquitoes around. Nicole maintains a private spiritual mentoring and teaching practice that currently operates online at www.nicolegoott.com.

References

Besant, Annie. *The Ancient Wisdom*. Adyar, India: The Theosophical Publishing House. 1994.

—*A Study in Consciousness. A contribution to the Science of Psychology*. Krotona: Theosophical Publishing House; Mansfield Centre, CT: Martino Publishing. 2010.

—*Dharma*. McAllister Editions. 2015.

Besant, Annie and Bhagaván Dás. *Sanātana Dharma*. Chennai: Theosophical Publishing House. 2000.

Bhagaván Dás. *The Science of Peace*. London and Benares: Theosophical Publishing Society. 1904.

Bstan-'dzin-rgya-mtsho. *Ethics for the New Millennium*. New York, New York: Riverhead Books. 1999.

Bstan-'dzin-rgya-mtsho, and Jeffrey Hopkins. *How to be compassionate – A Handbook for creating inner peace and a happier world*. New York, New York: Atria Paperback, a division of Simon & Schuster, Inc. 2011.

Chatterji, J.C. *Kashmir Shaivasim*. Albany, NY: State University of New York Press. 1986.

Easwaran, Eknath. *The Bhagavad Gita – Introduced and Translated by Eknath Easwaran*. Canada: Nilgiri Press. 2009.

Emoto, Masaru. Dr. *The Hidden Messages in Water*. Hillsboro, Oregon: Beyond Words Publishing, Inc. 2004.

Feuerstein, Georg. *Tantra, The Path of Ecstasy*. Boston, Massachusetts: Shambhala Publications, Inc. 1998.

Feuerstein, Georg. *The Encyclopedia of Yoga and Tantra*. Boston, Massachusetts: Shambhala Publications, Inc. 2011.

Ganczarek, J., Hünefeldt, T. & Olivetti Belardinelli, M. *From "Einfühlung" to empathy: exploring the relationship between aesthetic and interpersonal experience. Cogn Process* 19, 141–145 (2018). https://doi.org/10.1007/s10339-018-0861-x

Jaiswal, Yogini S. and Leonard L Williams. *A glimpse of Ayurveda – The forgotten history and principles of Indian traditional medicine,* 50–51. (2016). [Online] https://www.ncbi.nlm.nih.gov/pmc/articles/PMC5198827/

Lama Yeshe. *Introduction to Tantra. A Vision of Totality.* Boston, MA: Wisdom Publications.1987.

Lee, Bruce. *Striking Thoughts, Bruce Lee's Wisdom for Daily Living.* Tuttle Publishing, an imprint of Periplus Editions (HK) Ltd. 2016.

Leland, Kurt. *Music and The Soul. A Listener's Guide to Achieving Transcendent Musical Experience.* Charlottesville, VA: Hampton Roads Publishing Company, Inc. 2005.

Luskin, Fred. Forgive for Good. *A proven prescription for health and happiness.* New York, New York: Harper One, An Imprint of Harper Collins Publishers. 2003.

Luskin, F. (2004) "The Choice to Forgive", *Greater Good,* September 1, 2004. [Online] Available at https:// greatergood.berkeley.edu/article/item/the_choice_to_forgive (Accessed July 29, 2021).

Mallison, James and Mark Singleton. *Roots of Yoga.* Penguin Classics. 2017.

Paul, Russill. *The Yoga of Sound. Tapping the Hidden Power of Music and Chant.* Novato, CA: New World Library. 2004.

Roberts, Jane. *A Seth Book. The Nature of Personal Reality. Specific, practical techniques for solving everyday problems and enriching the life you know.* San Rafael, California: Amber-Allen Publishing. 1994.

Swami Satyananda Saraswati. *Nine Principle Upanishads: from the teachings of.* Bihar, India: Yoga Publications Trust. 2004.

Swami Venkatesananda. *Vasísthas's Yóga.* Albany, NY: State University of New York Press. 1993.

Taimni, I.K. *The Science of Yoga.* England: Quest Books. 1996.

***

Websites

Monier-Williams Sanskrit Dictionary Advanced (1899). [Online] https://www.sanskrit-lexicon.uni-koeln.de/scans/MWScan/2020/web/webtc2/index.php

Star Wars: Episode VI – Return of the Jedi (1983). Directed by Richard Marquand. Available at https://www.starwars.com/news/8-great-obi-wan-kenobi-quotes, August 14, 2019. (Accessed on May 19th, 2022).

Truth. (n.d.) In Oxford Languages and Google dictionary. Retrieved from https:www.google.com/seacrh?q=define+truth.

Universal. (n.d) In Merriam Webster online dictionary. Retrieved from https:www.merriam-webster/dictionary/universal.

Further Reading

Introduction

General information about the Vaiśeṣikasūtra and the five elements can be found on Wikipedia.

Accessed February 19, 2021 https://en.wikipedia.org/wiki/Vaiśeṣika_Sūtra

An excellent resource in general, and further information of timelines on important texts can be found in: Mallison, James and Mark Singleton. *Roots of Yoga.* Penguin Classics. 2017.

Chapter 2 – Cosmic Principles

Mishra, Kamalakar. *Kashmir Śaivism.* The Central Philosophy of Tantrism. Varanasi, India: Indica Books. 2011.

Chapter 5 – Water

Leland, Kurt. *Music and The Soul. A Listener's Guide to Achieving Transcendent Musical Experience.* Charlottesville, VA: Hampton Roads Publishing Company, Inc. 2005.

Chapter 7 – Mind

Feuerstein, Georg, with Brenda Feuerstein. *The Bhagavad Gita. A New Translation.* Boston, Massachusetts: Shambhala Publications, Inc. 2011.

Iyengar, B.K.S. *Light on the Yoga Sūtras of Patañjali.* Hammersmith, London: Harper Collins Publishers Limited. 2013.

Chapter 9 – Karma

Easwaran, Eknath. *The Bhagavad Gita – Introduced and Translated by Eknath Easwaran.* Canada: Nilgiri Press. 2009. (p.33)

***

Websites

www.theosophical.org

Bibliography

Chapter 1 – Subtle Bodies

Leland, Kurt. *Rainbow Body: A History of the Western Chakra System from Blavatsky to Brennan.* Ibis Press. 2016.

To understand the influence of the Theosophical Society, its teachings and transmission of ideas as a bridge between East and West, it is useful to examine this within the context of the Chakra system. I suggest as further reading on this subject, as well as the history of the Chakra system *Rainbow Body.*

Chapter 2 – Cosmic Principles

Frawley, David. *Ayurveda and the mind: the Healing of Consciousness.* Lotus Press. 2007.

The translation of each of the three gunas I utilized in this book are based upon the scholarship of Annie Besant. As these are possibly not as commonly known, and for students of Yoga and Ayurveda interested in further understanding or comparison, I refer the reader to the teaching of Dr. David Frawley.

Chapter 5 – Water

Mallison, James and Mark Singleton. *Roots of Yoga.* Penguin Classics. 2017.

During the course of research for this book, *Roots of Yoga* (Mallison and Singleton) proved to be an invaluable resource, as the authors are leaders in the field of scholarly authorship on a vast subject and philosophy. I believe that modern day students and practitioners of yoga will find this to be an enlightening source, in particular where the authors reveal new insights on some of the popular texts that are used and studied. This includes their comments on manuscripts such as the Yoga Sūtras of Patanjali, which the authors suggest be referenced differently than is commonly recognized at present. For readers interested in furthering their study of the subject, I recommend they consult the above-mentioned book.

Chapter 9 – Karma

Swami Krishnananada. *The Bṛhadāraṇyaka Upaniṣhad.* The Divine Life Society. [E-Book. No Date]

For readers interested in this Upanishad, in addition to a longer commentary on the particular aphorism mentioned in this book, I refer them to Swami Krishnananda's E-Book. The Divine Life Society offers this, as well as other commentaries on their website: www.swami-krishnananda.org.

Glossary

Abhiniveśāḥ – As a fear of dying and death, this has a double meaning. The first relates to the actual fear of dying and death over the course of a single lifetime. The second relates to a psycho-spiritual death and is the fear of the ego-personality dying. Both fears are rooted in the same core belief which is annihilation; that upon physical or spiritual death, the soul or spirit is completely extinguished. This is a root mental illusion and an obstacle on the path of personal liberation and freedom.

Ahamkāra – This is the principle called the "I-maker" which is the force of the ego. The "I-making" principle believes itself to be the real self which is what gives it power and energy.

Āsana – For the many millions of individuals that have explored the physical practices of yoga, āsana has the meaning of a physical posture that the body is shaped into through various movements. Āsana can also mean seat, and is the position that an individual places themselves in for a particular duration in the practice of meditation. This postural seat can include not only sitting but also lying down for instance, although sitting is more commonly associated with a posture for meditation. The postural practice found within the various expressions of yoga can all be seen from the perspective of preparing oneself for the deeper practices of yoga involving various contemplative and meditative exercises.

Asmitā – This is an illusion that clouds the lower mind whereby a belief or idea is held that the ego-personality is the real self. The illusion reinforces itself over and over, regenerating the inner picture of the false self as real and everlasting. This becomes a continual source of suffering, for as long as the illusion is maintained and believed in, the challenge of living from higher wisdom and guidance is drowned out.

Ātman – True Self signified by the capitalized "A." As the true Self, this could be thought of as something like the soul or spirit.

ātman – The false self signified by the lower case "a." The false self can be thought of as the part of the ego-personality that acts like a shadow, which is not only a blindspot of the individual, but also hides the true Self from others.

Avidyā – Vidyā means knowledge or to know. The opposite of this is not knowing, and sometimes translated as ignorance. In essence, it is the spiritual blindspot of not knowing encompassing the lack of knowing about the true nature of reality, the nature of the true Self, and that there is no true separation.

Ayurveda – Like earlier forms of medicine and healing, Ayurveda is a system that regards the person holistically as body, emotions, mind and spirit. The word itself is defined as the science or knowledge of life or a way of life. The knowledge of the system is reportedly over 5000 years old. One of the core principles is based on balancing the constitution of an individual by looking at the five elements and suggesting changes or modifications to all areas of life such as (but not limited to) diet and lifestyle.

Bindu – A single or central point in which not only is energy or a state of consciousness concentrated, it is also a focal point for a meditator to direct their attention toward.

Buddhi – Higher mind, the faculty of wisdom and discernment, the power to see things from a higher perspective. Not only is this a discernment of the higher mind beyond mental intelligence, it is a spiritual discernment leading one closer to alignment with one's dharma and the Source.

Chakra (Ćakra) – An energetic center within a subtle body. It can be described as a vortex of spinning energy, like a wheel that moves in perpetual motion. Each energy center has its own unique properties that contribute to the overall state of balance and functioning of an individual.

Dharma – Each individual has their own path in life, a purpose that drives the lessons and growth for each lifetime. There is often a great challenge in discovering what a person's unique life path is, as the individual navigates overcoming the conditioning adopted through social and family imprinting in favor of living in alignment with their true Self and true purpose.

Dveṣaḥ – Aversion to some form of experience whether that be a situation, a place, an object or a person, including some aspect of oneself. At its root, aversion arises from not liking something and or fear.

Jīva – Essence of a living being which includes an individual soul.

Jñānendriya – These are the senses by which experience is known. There are five knowledge senses that are related to the five physical organs. For example, we see physical reality with our physical eyes but we see inner reality with our inner eye.

Karmmendriya – These are the five organs of action in the physical body which include the mouth as speech and expression, the hands as grasping and manipulation of the physical environment, the feet as movement and locomotion of the body, the urinogenital system of elimination and procreation, and the system of digestion and elimination.

Kleśa – In essence, a klesha is a mental illusion, of which there are many, that creates an obstacle in the life of an individual. Since the illusion is generated in the mind, the only way to overcome the obstacle is to return to its source; the ideas and beliefs that give the illusion power. The Yoga Sutras of Patanjali enumerate five kleshas.

Mokṣa – Liberation in this sense is something that happens inwardly. Each step which brings an individual closer to knowing themselves – their true Self, is essentially following a path of inner liberation. Each step that strips away the no longer necessary forms of identity, bring about an inner change – an experience inwardly of freedom from all ideas of separation and annihilation. Each step represents a continual unfolding of this path of inner liberation. The only real and so-called "end" is the realization of the true nature of the Self and of Reality. But this is really just a beginning of a further unfolding of the soul's full potential. Another meaning of liberation is from the causes of rebirth. This essentially means that an individual is able to unwind the seeds of karma that they have brought with them into a current lifetime while simultaneously working fervently to live in such a way as to reduce or eliminate the creation of any new or further karma.

Pancha Jñānendriya – These are the five ways of knowing reality. *Pancha* is the numerical value of five. *Jñā* is the root word for knowing or to know. *Indriya* refers to the senses of perception.

Pancha Karmmendriya – These are the five action senses. Acting through the five senses to create reality has a causative effect. Thus, the senses could be thought of as the vehicles for being an agent of creating *karma,* the results of actions experienced in physical reality positively or negatively.

Parama Śiva – The ultimate source of reality, of all being, is represented as the ultimate or great Shiva.

Prāṇa – Everything that is consciousness has its own prana, which essentially means life force. It is the current of vitality that sustains each individual throughout their lifetime. Although it is never fully depleted, it does increase and decrease depending on life circumstances. High amounts of stress or illness for instance decrease life force whereas activities such as walking in nature increase life force.

Potluck – Potluck is a North American term where people are invited to share a meal together, each person contributing by bringing a prepared dish of their own. All the dishes combined make up the food to be collectively consumed.

Prāṇāyāma – If we look at this word in two parts we see it contains prana first, and yama second. As defined already, prana means life force. Yama is sometimes defined as restraint or constraint, but I tend to think of this as directing and focusing. Together, the two words imply a meaning of directing life force by applying one's focus, which would be the mind or attention. In Hatha Yoga, pranayama is experienced through various specialized breathing practices, each one having a particular focus. The outcome of each breath practice as a meditation, is an experience of a state of consciousness that usually differs from the ordinary waking experience. Aside from the meditation experiences, breathing practices can have a beneficial effect on the physical body.

Rāga – The principle by which reality is created through the force of desire and attachment, whether that be for a physical object, a situation, an experience of some kind, an individual or other sentient being such as a pet. Day to day, this appears in the more imperceptive form of pursuing what is "liked."

Sāṁkhya – This is one of the branches of a school of thought found within Indian philosophy. It is based on a principle of duality rather than a principle of oneness.

Saṃsāra – The cycle of rebirth, sometimes described as the repeated cycle of wandering from one lifetime to the next without knowing how to bring this repetition to an end. The events that keep the cycle or wheel spinning is the basis of karma – the causes and effects of countless choices.

Saṁskāra – A container holding the collection of thoughts, desires, wishes, fears – mental impressions. It is a storehouse of energy that can pass from one lifetime to the next, searching for the optimal conditions to empty out into physical reality and eventually ripen as a karmic event.

Śakti – Shakti is the co-equal counterpart to Shiva, representing the principle of the divine feminine in the Universe. Her power is the active form of creation, bringing something into physical being. Together, Shakti and Shiva represent the form of the universal and sacred divine couple; simultaneously co-equal yet two unique expressions joined by the same root connection – the Source. When brought together in ideal balance and harmony, they represent the joy and harmony of divine bliss.

Śiva – Shiva is the co-equal counterpart to Shakti, representing the principle of the divine masculine in the Universe. His power rests in the form of absorption, a state of divine bliss.

Sūtra – A sutra is written in the form of a collection of short statements or aphorisms which, when read as a whole, seamlessly weaves together a complete idea or philosophy. Each sutra itself can often be read individually, containing within itself a fully complete idea or thought, whereas a verse in a poem, for example, can lose the context and overall message that the author wishes to convey.

Tattva – A property of matter, down to the smallest particles. It is an essential essence that is that "thing."

Yoga – In general, this author understands Yoga to mean a process which moves an individual to closer union within themselves inwardly. The process gradually strips away anything that acts as an impediment to that union, with each step along the path akin to mini spiritual initiations. Each initiation is a challenge that must be overcome, learning the lesson that is intended for the individual. As the lesson is integrated, the individual progresses such that the development is an unfolding of the full potential and expression not as a separated identity, but rather a fully realized and blossoming Soul. Union is thus a movement toward balance, harmony and joy which are all expressions of the Soul. Yoga is as much an outer journey as it is an inner journey, and the ideal is to find a balance of both, bringing the outer and the inner into union.

Yogin – Traditionally, the gender of male yoga practitioner.

Yoginī – Traditionally, the gender of female yoga practitioner.

Yoga Nidra – The word nidra is typically translated as sleep. This is not the routine, nightly ritual of going to sleep, losing conscious awareness of the body and thoughts. Rather, yoga nidra is a practice of simultaneously staying consciously present and aware of the body that the practitioner has disengaged from thus allowing the body to rest, while remaining in relaxed and calm mental equipoise.

Index

Titles of Sanskrit texts appear in italics. Sanskrit names of persons and philosophies appear in IAST. All other Sanskrit terms appear anglicized without IAST. References to tables and illustrations appear in boldface.

journaling (exercise) 57–59, 67, 72–73, 127–128

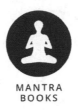

MANTRA
BOOKS

EASTERN RELIGION & PHILOSOPHY

We publish books on Eastern religions and philosophies. Books
that aim to inform and explore the various traditions that
began in the East and have migrated West.
If you have enjoyed this book, why not tell other readers by
posting a review on your preferred book site.

The Less Dust the More Trust
Participating in The Shamatha Project, Meditation and Science
Adeline van Waning, MD PhD
The inside-story of a woman participating in frontline
meditation research, exploring the interfaces of mind-practice,
science and psychology.
Paperback: 978-1-78099-948-7 ebook: 978-1-78279-657-2

I Know How To Live, I Know How To Die
The Teachings of Dadi Janki: A warm, radical, and life-
affirming view of who we are, where we come from, and what
time is calling us to do
Neville Hodgkinson
Life and death are explored in the context of frontier science
and deep soul awareness.
Paperback: 978-1-78535-013-9 ebook: 978-1-78535-014-6

Living Jainism
An Ethical Science
Aidan Rankin, Kanti V. Mardia
A radical new perspective on science rooted in intuitive
awareness and deductive reasoning.
Paperback: 978-1-78099-912-8 ebook: 978-1-78099-911-1

Ordinary Women, Extraordinary Wisdom
The Feminine Face of Awakening
Rita Marie Robinson
A collection of intimate conversations with female spiritual
teachers who live like ordinary women, but are engaged
with their true natures.
Paperback: 978-1-84694-068-2 ebook: 978-1-78099-908-1

The Way of Nothing
Nothing in the Way
Paramananda Ishaya
A fresh and light-hearted exploration of the amazing reality of
nothingness.
Paperback: 978-1-78279-307-6 ebook: 978-1-78099-840-4

Readers of ebooks can buy or view any of these bestsellers by
clicking on the live link in the title. Most titles are published
in paperback and as an ebook. Paperbacks are available in
traditional bookshops. Both print and ebook formats are
available online.

Find more titles and sign up to our readers' newslett er at
http://www.johnhuntpublishing.com/mind-body-spirit. Follow
us on Facebook at https://www.facebook.com/OBooks and
Twitter at https://twitter.com/obooks.